Perspectives on Later Life

Perspectives on Later Life

edited by

Peter R Day

Whiting & Birch Ltd

MCMXCIII

Published by Whiting & Birch Ltd,
Forest Hill, London SE23 3HZ

ISBN 1 871177 53 7 (cased)

Printed in England and the United States by Lightning Source

Contents

Acknowledgements

We are most grateful to Wendy Clarke of the University of Newcastle-upon-Tyne and to Dorothy Buckley and Rosie Woolley of the Centre for Research in Social Policy at Loughborough University of Technology. Their all round efficiency and hard work have been invaluable.

Introduction

Peter Day

There is no shortage of research on later life which is relevant to social policy and social work and social care practice. There are examples of excellent facilities available to improve the life satisfaction of older people where research, practice wisdom and progressive policies have been linked in creative ways (Payne, 1989a). But there is some way to go in providing social care which recognises the importance of responding to consumer choice in the light of research on later life. Ideally residential and day care services should help their users to obtain the best quality of life of which they are capable. It should be a better life, according to the Wagner Committee (Wagner, 1988) than would be available in any other environment.

Despite great hopes that the Wagner Committee report would lead to improvements, residential care seems to be no more of a positive choice than it was in 1988 and at least one commentator has written of a time of darkness in residential care. Certainly reports of the problems revealed in the 1990s and the abuses in children's homes have been depressing. It has been pointed out that there have been sixty major reports about the spectrum of residential care since 1946 which have drawn attention to the need to improve staff training. But if the same old excuses for poor and abusive practice are being used in 1993 why has there been such consistent failure to recognise the obvious and to act on it? There seems to be a marked failure to value and recognise the needs of care staff. To recruit people to provide care for those who may be vulnerable, disturbed and frail individuals in all age groups and to leave carers without adequate guidance, support and training invites the problems we know exist in residential care. The provision of adequate professional support for staff would seem to be beset by both organisational and resource problems.

The motivation to produce this book was based on concern to try to combat the continuing apparent inadequacies in the quality and quantity of education, training and professional supervision available to students and staff working, or preparing to work, in residential and day care services for older people. In particular many people who were concerned shared the editor's concern that some education and training courses were still (in recent years) using out dated material and that many care workers felt unsupported and lacked adequate supervision. Factors ranging from lack of teaching on recent research, failure to adopt modern methods of care, the poor image of residential care and inadequate consultation with carers all contribute to the failings evident in residential care.

Radical changes in attitudes are needed to make an impact on these endemic problems and this provides a main thrust in this book.

Some of the ideas which were around when the proposal to re-examine research and practice was first mooted are discussed below. A major impetus came with the sad events of 1990 in the residential care of children and young people. Prior to this there had been numerous reports which had consistently drawn attention to the need to improve staff training in residential care. Pin down, relating to young people in care, was comparable to what we were thinking about in relation to the care of older people. Research and theory were being misapplied and basic principles of care seemed to be ignored. Until very recently ageing has been seen as either an extremely negative fact of life or the absolute opposite, a period of serene contentment and satisfaction. It is unrealistic to ignore the anger and pain involved at this stage of development and it would be inaccurate to ignore the deprivation and disadvantages experienced by many people in later life. Some older people do have a poor quality of life but, in recent years, there has been more awareness that some views of old age are unnecessarily negative. Our concern in this book is to take a realistic and balanced view of later life and to emphasise certain key themes:

- that later life is part of a life path or, the phrase commonly used, life span development;
- that individuals need to be understood within their cultural and social context.

One reason for looking at life span development–the process of growing older–in cultural and social context is that it should aid understanding of attitudes which are widespread and which affect carers and health and social services staff. The policies which affect people in later life and their families are, of course based on these dominant attitudes. The growing numbers of older people in the population are frequently referred to as a burden, or social problem. If sensitive care is to be provided the impact of such attitudes needs to be appreciated–not least on older people's views of themselves. Social structures do not treat people equally. Groups of people are commonly distinguished by criteria such as physique and size, ethnicity, sex, abilities and disabilities and age. These kinds of criteria are used to rank people to form different kinds of hierarchies on the basis of access to resources. People with access to resources usually have power or the ability to enforce their will on others. Powerful people control the decision making about how resources will be distributed. Those with power have more control over and access to economic processes. They have more goods and services as well as decision making power. By contrast the poor have little money and limited ability to get the resources they need and they experience higher rates of social isolation, unemployment, ill health and crime. Membership of minority groups (for example, very old people) increases the likelihood that access to resources will be limited. Structural inequalities clearly have an effect on people's abilities to exercise freedom. There are clearly material gains for some citizens which result from social injustice and this poses individuals with moral dilemmas about their wider social obligations. In recent years the dominant philosophy of the property owning democracy has dealt with the problem of inequality by regarding social justice as a fantasy or mirage. Individuals have a moral obligation to look after themselves and their families but beyond this no one should expect help from anyone else. This view of social structure was summed up as follows. 'There is no such thing as society, only individuals and their families'. Family responsibility and individual self reliance are thus the central ideas of the contemporary orthodoxy although it is recognised that there are some people who are not self-sufficient because of personal inadequacy or adverse circumstances. For less fortunate people, social services are provided if genuine need is demonstrated. This is only a brief reference to the property owning democracy, but it is important to observe that this philosophy is not free of ambiguity and inconsistency, both in theory and practice. It is important to appreciate also that there are other philosophies based on different values and therefore having different views on social justice, individual freedom and responsibility, and the notion of community.

In keeping with the philosophy just outlined, current attitudes to old age are mainly influenced by the notion of economic productivity. Individuals are valued on the basis of what they produce and elderly people are generally thought of as unproductive. It has been pointed out that this is used to explain or justify the conditions in which elderly people are expected to live. There are, of course, problems in linking the stereotyped view of old age with the individualistic ethic which supports and perpetuates wide disparities in the incomes and living standards found in contemporary society. Not all elderly people are impoverished and this fact may be leading to a change in attitudes. It is not our intention to dwell unnecessarily on negative features of residential care and later life which have been recognised in the popular press as well as professional journals over the years. We do need to recognise them however since they are a large part of our subject matter. Ageist attitudes are based on fear and as we have seen, like racism and sexism, they deprive people of power and influence. These attitudes are important because they affect the way in which older people see themselves, how they are seen by others and the way services are provided (or not provided) for them. The problems with ageism are that it is largely based on fiction and it affects members of the caring professions as well as the general public. Some of these myths are dealt with in this book. The assumptions that ill-health, senility, inflexibility, mental deterioration, isolation, misery and unproductivity are all characteristics of later life and are all questionable. It is correct only to say that they apply to a small proportion of older people. Old age is not necessarily a time when life is dominated by sickness and disability. There are positive aspects to growing older and later life is for many people a productive and happy part of the life span. An increasing proportion of people from ethnic minority groups in the United Kingdom are now reaching later life. They may have special needs: their minority status of both race and age combine to make them vulnerable to deprivation and stress. There are stresses connected with having been immigrants to this country. Some people who came in as dependents are not eligible for income support and their relative poverty leads to stress which is exacerbated by poor housing and poor quality or patchy health and social services. Some of them, like some indigenous people, may fear ending up in residential care. It is becoming clearer that the strong, caring and all-embracing extended black family is a false idea: it is incorrect to assume that all members of ethnic minorities have comprehensive support from their families and communities. This is slowly being recognised by voluntary and statutory agencies, especially in areas where minority groups have been able to make representations about their needs.

The starting point of Chapter 1 is the understanding that people in later life need to be thought of, not as a separate category of 'elderly person' but as people in a particular part of the life cycle and in a social context which has demographic and political implications. This implies that the elderly person's position in the community requires a particular practice approach aimed at enabling them to live in a satisfying way. Three aspects of social work in field, residential and day care settings are considered:

- assessment of needs and evaluation of services;
- the decision about intervention;
- the nature of intervention and the client's social systems.

The chapter concludes by reviewing the inadequacy of many social work theories and of the organisation of services.

Chapter 2 reviews some psychological perspectives on later life. It develops the idea that ageing is the process of life time development. Later life is a stage in the process which is followed by death. As individuals become more aware of ageing, usually from the third decade, the recognition of time passing is usually a matter of sadness. Alongside the feelings of loss and apprehension however most people are able to express feelings of satisfaction at growing older. The relevance of research to understanding reactions to change and how people adapt in later life are reviewed in this chapter.

Chapter 3 also looks at later life as a stage in the life span and develops the idea mentioned earlier that quality of life is strongly influenced by the individual's position and role in the social structure. It argues that the individual needs to be understood in the cultural and social context if stereotyped and incorrect images are to be avoided. Ageing is not necessarily a social problem but some individuals encounter personal problems of ill health and disability as they grow older, and they may have special needs as a result. Social relationships change with advancing age and social isolation can be a difficulty for elderly people–for example, for people who are single or widowed and who have no other surviving relatives or friends. The chapter thus underlines the diversity of experience in later life and on this basis discusses the implications for social policy and social care.

Chapter 4 discusses the types of housing in which older people live and problems which arise for them in comparison with people at earlier stages of the life span. Older people are more likely to be poor, disabled, badly housed and widowed. These disadvantages have an effect on the ability of some people to live independently. The decisions that face people in later life and the choices they have are bound by experiences, expectations and external resources and by individual personality and psychological resources. The chapter discusses the development of personal and social care services which should enable people to remain in their own homes with necessary support or make a positive choice to move to special housing or residential care. The many complex factors, including stereotyping, which influence the quality of services, are discussed in this chapter.

Prejudiced beliefs are held about people who are seen as different on account of their gender, age, disability or ethnic origin. Racist, disablist, ageist or sexist attitudes are attributed to those who have the power to turn their prejudice into acts of discrimination or unfair treatment. Discrimination can be conscious or unconscious and operates at individual and institutional levels. Thus individual or direct racism, for example, occurs when a person treats people unfairly because of their ethnic origins. Institutional or indirect racism found in organisations or services is more common and happens in a variety of ways. It may happen by default in that the needs of people from ethnic minorities are not taken into account. It may be seen when the catering facilities for people are based on what is usually eaten by the white majority. It is apparent when people have difficulties in gaining access to health and social services. Indirect racism is seen where people in positions of power base their decisions on racist stereotypes or assumption. For example, it may be assumed, incorrectly, that black and ethnic minority families care for their own members and do not require support services. It is sometimes hard to recognise how stereotyped attitudes affect thinking and behaviour. Issues of gender are embedded in residential care and many carers are women. Among residents, women outnumber men and low standards of care and privacy may reflect this. In this book attention is given to issues of stereotyping and unfair dissemination and ageist attitudes are challenged.

Among the stereotype which need to be examined are those which suggest that later life automatically involves physical and mental deterioration and that the elderly personality is a fixed and unchanging entity. These widely held assumptions lead to gloomy and fatalistic views about the limits of medical and psychological help for older individuals experiencing problems in adjustment. Some older people not only have to come to terms with loss of function and capacity but may also have to deal with the insensitivity of their carers. It has been estimated that up to 10% of people aged over 65 years suffer from confused mental states and this has a variety of effects. An individual may become disorientated in time and space; there may be changes in behaviour resulting from inability to control impulses and failure to conform socially, loss of memory occurs and can be very anxiety provoking, and people may wander or their behaviour appears to be aimless. These changes may be very worrying for the individual concerned and for those around him or her as he or she observes him or herself coping less and less successfully. Such special difficulties in adjustment and ways of dealing with them are covered in Chapter 5.

The process of ageing is associated with loss of various kinds–loss of paid occupation, loss of friends and relatives, and physical and mental changes leading to disability and loss of control over one's own life. Loss is inevitable throughout life and is encountered frequently as people grow older and by carers and workers with older people. The subject matter of Chapter 6 raises problems for most people and in studying loss and bereavement this has to be taken into account: it significantly affects the conduct of research on these subjects. There is now quite a vast literature on dying and grief however and this chapter refers to a range of theoretical and research orientations. Sociological approaches to dying complement medical and psychological research. Perspectives which have special relevance for care workers include life span development, attachment theory and interactionist approaches in sociology. The implications of research on counselling methods and outcomes will be considered.

The concluding chapters of the book are concerned with people involved in caring for older people, some of whom are themselves in the later part of the life path. Research is now indicating more about the circumstances of the growing group of people–over one million women and men–who have given up much of their lives to look after disabled and elderly dependents. This group of people have been described as a forgotten army and are the subject of

Chapter 7.

In the last chapter the position of formal carers and the importance of staff training and development will be discussed. The Wagner committee referred to earlier argued that a fundamental change is needed in public attitudes to residential care and its place in health and social services. It should be seen as part of the pattern of community care. These ideas provoke complex questions about the central relationship between quality of care and staff morale. This is examined in the final chapter. It is a challenging topic–the recommendations of official enquiries, like the effect of most research, are adopted selectively and often irrationally. At the beginning of this introduction I referred to many examples of progressive caring practices where workers are able to implement relevant research and theory. It is important to underline this recognition.

In writing this book then we seek to be positive and to look for hope for improvement where it is needed. Ideas are given about the kinds of contributions which readers can make and the book aims to make good some of the deficiencies of earlier education and training and to draw attention to modern approaches in social gerontology. It is addressed to carers, staff, voluntary workers, elderly people themselves and to managers and trainers too. It is hoped that readers will have the confidence to challenge poor practice based on out of date research, theory and hide bound ideas, to constantly question theoretical fashions and snobbery and to recognise and reaffirm much that is good in their practice

One

New understandings of later life: practice and service implications

Malcolm Payne

THE EXPERIENCE OF LATER LIFE

My mother died recently, aged 81, having lived alone for more than 25 years after the death of my father. In the last few years, she needed help. She was well-provided for by the social services department (Harrow), with home helps three times a day, seven days a week. Attempts had been made to provide her with meals on wheels ('not as good as they have in hospital,' she told me); there were aids and adaptations to the house; the Red Cross supplied a commode. A district nurse visited weekly.

She was frightened of falling; staunchly independent, she would never ask for anything and fought against being dependent and receiving help. She resisted the home help service, and whenever I made helpful suggestions, she would suspiciously ask if I knew this as a social worker (and so it was unacceptable information). Next door, a retired teacher 'was just like a daughter to me', looked in every day, dealt with several crises, and responded to calls for help at any hour of the day or night. In a serious disaster, another neighbour, a young man who had never met my mother, rallied round to help pick her up from the floor.

These personal experiences of later life in my family are at the front of my mind in offering this account of social work with older people because they force me to start from life as it is experienced by people that we call 'clients'. There are three important points to make. First, later life is experienced by people living through it not as something different called 'old age' but as part of a continuing existence. Second, relationships and humanity are still present, whether offered through official care or through neighbours and friends; later life is not just an experience, but it is a *social* experience. Third, there are special things to cope with in later life - infirmity, disability, dependence perhaps - but these fall within the continuity of experience and the social pattern of earlier years.

SOCIAL CARE AND THE EXPERIENCE OF LATER LIFE

The continuity of our development into later life, and the consequences of this for how we must understand the theory and practice of social care work is the major point of this chapter. I argue that we must understand clients in later life within their social and personal backgrounds, with their existing personal psychology and attitudes transferred into a new situation. To put it in the traditional formulation of psychosocial social casework (Hollis and Woods, 1981), it is the person and the situation that we must understand. We must take the very real physical, psychological and personal consequences of ageing into account and place them within our contextualised understanding of the whole life of older people. In particular, we should not let the 'typical' characteristics of old age define the whole life within which we are working.

Our society creates social structures and assumptions which tend to define how we think about people in later life. For example, men usually die before women, leaving a larger population of older women who have been in partnerships during their life, and our services and way of living are constructed according to the implications of this fact.

How are we to see the role of social care services within this experience of life and 'later life'? The first point to make, thinking again of continuity, is that much care occurs within the patterns of existing social relationships or links which arise naturally in the development of an older person's life experience. Insofar as care is 'social' it should be organised as part of those existing relationships, since it should be a counterpart of those links.

The second point is that 'care' needs, in my view, to be de-emphasised within social care; the emphasis should be on the social. In many respects care is both routine and requires personal commitment. Parker (1981), in a ground-breaking paper, has emphasised that much of what is offered to people as 'care' is relatively routine, but nonetheless skilled, 'tending'; attendance to their wishes and needs on a consistent basis. *Social* care emphasises mutuality of responsibility and involvement. Thus, while we can prepare for, plan and 'deliver' tending services, we can only offer 'social care' by involvement in the pattern of life, the network of social relationships and an acknowledgement and understanding of the social environment which people in later life experience. This is true of our work with all clients, but is worth emphasising about people in later life, because of the length of time during which their pattern of life and relationships has been built up and the devastation caused by disrupting such ingrained patterns.

The changing social situation and changing experience of life might alter our responses to people in older life and the services they require. For example, the modern pattern whereby families are more widely spread, a high proportion of women work and there are more single parent families with a woman as head of household and sole or main wage earner than was once the case has implications now for what family care is available to people in later life who need care. In the future, it will have implications for how the present generation of people in middle life as they grow older will expect to live and the networks for care that they will have available.

AVOIDING CATEGORISING IDEAS

Since I have argued that we should see social care work with those in later life in its changing social context, it is important to avoid getting hung up on ideas which categorise 'old people' in ways which limit the flexibility of our understanding and work.

First, we should beware of seeing something intrinsically different about 'old age', because of the medical problems covered by the professionally defined speciality of 'geriatrics', because of the social policy category of 'services to old people', and through the social assumption that something happens at 'retirement' and through the social consequences of ageing which creates a category of people called 'the elderly' who must be treated differently in some way from others. I regard these categorisations as mere administrative conveniences, and like many conveniences, they may lead us to risk over-simplification.

Of course, many people in later life suffer from a deterioration in physical functioning; there are changes in eyesight, hearing and ability to move around. In eyes, for example, the pupil size reduces, so that less light can enter the eye, muscles lose their control of lens thickness, the lens yellows, darkens and grows larger and cannot focus on near objects, optic nerves lose cells and reduce the amount of detail that can be seen, and the transparent part of the eye produces more 'floaters', the harmless shapes we sometimes see across our vision (Weale, 1989). These changes may affect the older person's freedom to act and live as they would wish. Hipkiss and Bittles (1989) summarise some of the theories which try to account for these physical changes, which include the idea that bodies are wearing out, or conversely that they are accumulating damaging poisons. Alternative ideas try to explain ageing not by looking at changes in the whole body, but by identifying changes in the way cells and molecules work in later life.

I have indicated the range of these ideas and the detail of one area of physical change in later life (in the eyes) to draw attention to the need for social workers to recognise that physical deterioration is a reality and must be dealt with realistically, so that people can be helped to deal with consequent disabilities and accept the limitations that they must accept. Even though these changes are fairly general, and perhaps because they are fairly general, we must guard against the assumption that natural changes require or permit us to treat older people with less respect, involvement and commitment.

Another idea which unreasonably categorises people in later life is 'disengagement'. Disengagement theory sees later life as a progress away from involvement in wide social contacts towards a more limited set of experiences - there is supposed to be a loss of interest in the world, a decrease in activity and a limitation of social contacts.

On the surface, you could see this in my mother. When she stopped work, she carried on with the various organisations she was a member of and took up one or two new ones. Over the years, however, these fell away, until her daily round was of a visit to local shops (rather than the town), business carried out by letter, and contact only with the occasional visiting relatives and a very few neighbours. But to accept this surface impression was not to know her. In fact, she knew more about what was going on in the family than I did, who was constantly about in the world. She was constantly interested in my sons, loved receiving letters and visits from them and was fascinated by the lifestyle of my cousins in the USA and Australia. She remained an incredibly amusing raconteur about events in the neighbourhood and within her past life.

What limited her was her increasing immobility due to arthritis, and a certain impatience with her slowness, a wish not to be a burden to anyone else, and therefore not to parade her weaknesses by needing help in the local shops and above all, in the later years, her fear of falling. I was impressed by her nurse and social worker, who, after a crisis, concentrated their efforts on her mobility and her fear, because these were the crucial elements of her limitations, and they gave her an extra summer of reasonable security and happiness before problems closed in again.

My personal experience, and everyone's knowledge of the activity and involvement of older people all around them, gives the lie to the assumption that disengagement is inevitable. The fact that it happens arises from the reality of how old age may affect us. It also arises from how we all respond to those realities of later life. Our society so much excludes older people from participation, by its impatience and lack of consideration, and by its concentration on economic and social expectations which are centred on younger people. For example, social provision tends to be concentrated on those who have the capacity to pay high prices for packaged entertainment, and provides less where there is no profit to be made. Older people then have to rely on special provision or provision which is not targeted to their interests. The special provision implies a ghetto, and may imply dependence on charitable or social welfare provision, rather than contributing to an independent and participative delivery of services.

So the false assumption of disengagement goes alongside the creation of dependence on social provision, and is more a product of how, as a society, we choose to respond to people in later life thus forcing older people into a particular response to us. I have often wondered, for example, why we provide limited social opportunities for brief parts of the day for unstimulating activities and institutional cooking in ghetto day centres, when we could facilitate attendance at the local pub for more typical entertainment, involvement in a wider clientele, a more culturally acceptable meal.

Another idea which can be inappropriately categorising is that old age is a phase in a 'life cycle'. This concept is useful because it emphasises continuity in our lives and seeks to value every stage of the life equally.

However, there are problems with the life cycle. First, it implies the circularity of the process of living, and this tends, in my view, to restrict the life cycle to growing up, family life and the reproduction of children (who become the beginning of a new cycle). This tends to push old age out of the cycle, which has been completed before old age is reached. Another problem with seeing life as a cycle, is that in some senses later life can be assumed to be like a return to childhood, in which dependence and need for care is an important aspect, when we should be emphasising the links to adulthood and self-dependence.

Second, the idea of the life cycle still tends to emphasise childhood and the family as the starting points and centre of life, with old age at the end. By treating life in marked phases, it fails to make clear the way in which ageing is a part of every aspect of life, forming more and more significant trails which lead into our later life in chronological terms.

Third, most significant of all, talking about the life cycle or life course still centres ageing about the experience of individuals or groups of old people. It fails to emphasise the fact that later life is socially determined by how we treat and respond to elderly people and how our society constructs expectations and the contexts in which later life is lived.

Laczko and Phillipson (1991) emphasise the significance of the 'political economy' model of understanding later life, which allows us to take into account this important social aspect of understanding ageing. In this view, how people live in later life is 'socially constructed' by their position in the social structure and by economic and social factors which form that social structure, including especially the effect of factors which may lead to discrimination against some or all older people. This includes racism, sexism and ageism.

Ageism reflects the marginalisation of the whole group of people in later life through social processes which have emphasised the definition of a group of people labelled 'elderly' and the construction of them as different and dependent. Townsend (1986) argues that the state plays an important role in raising dependency and lowering status as a consequence. More than one of these discriminations may apply to any group or to any individual, and none of the discriminations can be assumed to be any more important than another, but one may be felt to be more important by particular clients.

It is important to realise, too, older people may be disadvantaged by their own assumptions: a simple example was my mother's lack of preparedness to use my experience as a social worker, because, in part, of her assumptions about the competence of a male to offer caring help.

SOCIAL CONTEXTS JUSTIFYING SPECIAL CONSIDERATION

If we are to consider older people in a social setting therefore, we should examine a variety of social aspects of their life, in just the same way as we would investigate those of a child or adult who become clients. We also need to examine them on a historical basis. When social workers undertake social histories of children, they often concentrate on the early 'stepping stones', and parental relationships and involvement with the child, since these are an important aspect of the child's personal history. With offenders, we look at the development of offending behaviour, with mentally ill people the development of the behaviour which is diagnosed as forming the illness.

In the case of elderly people, however, we are concerned not with a particular problematic form of behaviour, but with a whole life experience and the current situation which has arisen from it. With older people, there is a great deal more of life experience and circumstances to be taken into account than there is with younger people. In one case I dealt with, for example, I was struck by the relationship difficulties for an old lady's son which arose from the fact that she had left his father when the son was young to live with another man. When the new husband, 40-odd years later, died, her original husband moved back in for a further period of married life of more than 15 years before he too died, raising the need for care and lack of support that I was faced with.

Social workers need to explore the complexities of relationships over many years and their impact on the present situation as well as the social contexts which form the experiences of later life for many older people. As always in social work, we must also examine any factors which are likely to involve discrimination including especially gender and ethnic factors, disability and ageism.

It is only possible here to outline the importance of many of these social contexts; some of them are dealt with more fully later in this book. The point of doing so is to emphasise both the range of social contexts which it is right to explore when dealing with people in later life, and also the way in which these contexts grow from previous life experience and reflect exactly the same social issues as we all face throughout life. Social work practice requires us to understand in our assessments and interventions the impact of these social contexts on our clients; before we can examine social work theory and practice, therefore, we must see what issues are likely to face us in dealing with people in later life.

Employment, retirement and activity

Older people generally do not have paid employment; indeed in the 1980s there has been a movement to earlier unemployment through retirement of people in later life. Services and income support may not have caught up with the effects of early retirement in many occupations (Laczko and Phillipson, 1991). Some writers (e.g. Handy, 1989) have argued that the pattern of employment is changing, so that more people have periods of working intermittently for themselves and from home as adjuncts to smaller industries, rather than as mass employees of large industrial complexes for life. However, though they may not be paid, everyone is inevitably employed, whether at voluntary work, at personal endeavours of some kind, whether doing the gardening or the washing up, or personal development activities, or in some leisure or educational activity. Social workers dealing with older people will need to examine how the latter occupy themselves, and their attitude towards that occupation. That attitude and the extent to which an older person is satisfied with their activities will reflect their social expectations and the attitudes of people in the community around them. If their friends expect a largely leisured life based on the home, then this may be acceptable, and wider activities can be seen as imaginative and developmental. If their friends expect more - perhaps continuing involvement in their profession - a home-based existence forced on people by financial difficulties or by illness may come to seem frustrating and inadequate.

The psychological and interpersonal consequences of changes in retirement patterns may raise many difficulties for older people and their wider families. There is a conventional assumption, for example, perhaps fostered by Townsend's early research (1963), that in working class communities the experience of having a retired husband at home 'under their feet' was frustrating to wives and marital relationships deteriorated.

Phillipson (1987) compares retired car workers, miners and architects and shows that the pattern varies according to the social patterns in the community concerned. Retired car workers, living in a community of young families, were more isolated, whereas for miners in a close-knit community retirement was a communal experience, and architects and their wives carried on with part-time patterns of involvement in career and life outside the home. This sort of research emphasises the need for social workers to avoid taking for granted assumptions about social patterns, and look instead at the actual social forces at work on the people that they deal with. These may offer strengths that we often assume are not present.

Social workers may need to help older people consider and come to a realistic view about their work and retirement experience. An individual may be bitter about their enforced early exit from work, for example. They may blame their own inadequacies, or the employer's policies, or the way they were treated by particular managers. The important thing is to come to a realistic appraisal and an appropriate psychological response to that appraisal. This may not require 'acceptance' in the sense of acquiescence in what has happened to them. So, poor employment and social policies may justify a response such as campaigning for change, or seeking additional recompense.

Social workers concerned with the development of community services can also consider helping retiring people into appropriate community and social activities or new work patterns. Since traditional modes of retirement did not include such activities, or only expected them from middle class rather than working class people, considerable help may be needed to identify and develop ways in which retired people can create interesting new activities in their retirement and complete the 'rite of passage' into new social groupings. Since many people, perhaps especially men, gain their social contacts through work life, this may be an important community work strategy.

Income and income maintenance

In order to live, we have to have an income. The conventional way of gaining income for an adult is to work and receive payment for it, but, of course, there are many exceptions to this pattern. We have seen how in recent decades it has been the assumption that people in later life will be unemployed through 'retirement', and this leads to the acceptance that they will need to have an income through other means. This is achieved through transfer payments (mainly the state pension schemes and income support) from the present working population to those who are unable to work and through deferred wages (pensions funded by payments by individuals during their working lifetimes). The experience of many older people is reflected in the interviews in Bytheway's (1989, p.102) small study in Wales that '...later life has been characterised by a continuing struggle to cope with chronic disabilities and to maintain the supply of basic resources.'

The adequacy of today's financial provision for older people is the focus of considerable debate, considered in some detail by Blaikie and Macnicol (1989). Fundamentally the debate turns on how you interpret the comparisons between existing pension provision and average wages or typical incomes in families.

For the social worker concerned about individual families, there will be two crucial issues. The first is whether all the possible and appropriate benefits have been claimed from public or private social security systems. It is equally important to ensure, nowadays, that people have considered schemes for taking money out of the house they live in by some of the mortgage schemes that are available (although there are problems) as it is to ensure that they have claimed all their income support entitlements.

The second area is more complex and needs considerable skill, but it has the benefit of involving older people in debate and decisions about their needs. This is to explore the extent to which people are satisfied with the income they receive, comparing it with their lifetime experience. Many older people now have lived through war and social and economic deprivation and see many of the material benefits of their present situation in comparison with their past. It is also necessary to look at the environment that they live in and the social comparisons that they make, together with their expectations and wishes about the kind of life that they wish to lead. Thus, for example, the pensioners who lost their pensions through the Maxwell scandal may not in practice be any worse off than many ordinary people living on state pensions, but they will be in social milieux and have had expectations and interests that have prepared them for a rather different lifestyle in retirement.

Housing and environment

One of the important financial pressures for older people is maintaining their housing, but it is also an important social issue, because it raises the issue of whether housing for older people should be different from that for other adults, and perhaps segregated in some way or whether it should be integrated into ordinary housing (Butler with Tinker, 1983). The Wagner Committee on residential care (Wagner, 1988) argues that there should be a 'spectrum' of housing and services which should not necessarily go together. This would range from people living in their own homes or with other people in their families, through sheltered housing with minimal services, sheltered housing with a wider range of care services available, and traditional residential and nursing homes, with residents living communally, and with extensive services being provided on the premises.

Most people in later life live in ordinary accommodation, but while this may be integrated and socially desirable for the people concerned, there are problems. If they have stayed in their family home, it may be too large or in other ways unsuited to their needs. One problem may be that it has poor insulation and heating, and schemes to insulate older people's houses have been initiated. Special help may be needed with fuel. Since retirement may last for 20-30 years, the social identity of the area may have changed, creating social isolation. Sometimes problems arise from the environment of an older person's house. There may be fear from the possibility of crime against the house or the person, difficulty in getting to shops, poor social facilities and an unpleasant urban landscape. In rural areas, isolation and poor transport facilities can equally well lead to isolation. So can moving to a retirement area. Karn (1977) studied a group of these and found that it was the improved environment that they sought, becoming aware later of the advantages in improved social life in living in a retirement community. Generally, she found that the move worked well.

Since the 1950s, government has attempted to encourage the growth of sheltered housing and sometimes with associated services (Butler et al., 1983). These provide good support but may be isolating and expensive for the benefits that they confer. During the 1980s, there has been a large expansion in residential and nursing home provision in the private sector, which has had financial advantages over public provision through 'perverse' incentives identified by the Audit Commission (1986). This report, and other expressed concern, has led to the development of government policies to promote community care through the National Health Service and Community Care Act, 1990. There has also been a recent growth in ownership of housing, and

Evandrou and Victor (1989) show that people who own their own houses have better material advantages and more flexibility of action, are more healthy and make more use of services; this was not entirely connected with social class differences.

For the social worker, the links between care, housing and environment suggest again the importance of evaluating not only how clients see care needs, but how they view their housing and environment. This is inevitably related to the views of those around them. For example, Sinclair (1988a) shows that few older people want to go into residential care, and that family attitudes are an important feature of decisions to use residential care. In spite of attempts to create rational models of service provision through community care plans in each area, the attempt to shift resources from residential to community care will be more affected by such attitudes.

Education, leisure and social stimulation

Education and learning is an important part of later life. I make this point first, because there is a tendency among younger people to assume that learning tends to reduce with age - we talk of habit, or obstructiveness of behaviour, or stubbornness. However, older people must still learn to manage life and to retain interests and concerns about it exactly as everyone else must. In fact they adapt to substantial changes in the way their life is lived - the loss of friends, of social contexts, changes in relationship with their families and social expectations of them as older people.

Abrams (1989) comments on information from the General Household Survey that older people participate little in sports and activities, but rather more in social activities such as going to the cinema, outings to events or historic buildings and going to clubs and societies. However, many educational and leisure activities (e.g. aerobics, evening classes) can be and are adapted for older people. In the same way that younger people would be encouraged to experiment and expand their educational horizons, social workers should encourage and enable this for older people, whether in the community or in residential care, and in community development work should seek to develop educational opportunities.

In this connection, Groombridge (1989, p.178) draws attention to the right to education throughout life and quotes the United Nations' *Declaration of Human Rights:* 'Everyone has the right to education...Education shall be directed to the full development of the human personality'. Pilley (1990) in a survey of projects for older people throughout Europe shows how older people can be initiators and doers, rather than passive recipients of education and gives examples of information projects run by and for older people, self-help educational programmes up to university level, schemes for voluntary work and other community activity organised by older people and international exchange projects.

One important educational process can be used in therapeutic ways by social workers, and this is the idea of developing reminiscence work with older people, where they review experiences in an organised way, designed to integrate their life experiences with present reality, and assist in retaining contact with reality (Coleman, 1986). Marshall (1990, p.76) suggests that this can be particularly useful in working with older people who suffer from dementia, and proposes 'life story' books such as those used with children to help them see their life in context and remember important aspects of previous life. Many older people enjoy and value looking back on their lives and experiences, so this therapeutic activity can be interesting to and appreciated by many of them. This work may also be done in both residential, day and community settings.

Personal, family and social relationships

One of the most important aspects of social work is concern for personal, family and social relationships of clients. With people in later life, there are some aspects of these that are unusual. Many older people will be suffering from some degree of loss; they are more likely than people at other times of life to have experienced bereavement recently, and, as Rochford (1985, p.107) puts it, the loss of a longstanding partner 'encounters all those other earlier losses' which a person may have experienced. Bytheway (1989, p.103) in his small study of Welsh steelworkers and their families comments that '...it is the deaths of others that lead people into a sense of being old. Doris in 1987 is living alone, feeling incapable, unneeded and vulnerable and wondering why she should struggle on'. This quotation indicates the importance of bereavement in the felt capacity to manage other aspects of life in old age. There may be social losses, arising from moving from an established home into specialised housing or residential or nursing care.

Social workers will also be conscious of the range of informal supports in the older person's life. My mother had a variety of these, and even isolated people may have several informal connections. Wenger (1984) has shown how networks of care can extend into community and family links, although the networks that particular elderly people will have vary widely. One of the useful purposes of tapping the elderly person's own network is to find help for the less personal aspects of caring. Organised schemes for support have been arranged. Robinson (1991) for example, describes the supportive possibilities of respite care schemes which help full-time carers gain some relief on a regular or occasional basis from the burdens of caring. Such burdens include loss of employment and financial costs, social costs in that links with friends may be lost, emotional psychological and physical coasts (Allen et al., 1983).

Most of these burdens will fall on members of the family, however, firstly on the spouse or long-time partner, and then on sons, daughters and occasionally on more distant relatives. Thus, the extent to which older people can get help from non-official sources will depend on family and social links. The requirements of caring will also have a major impact on family relationships, and have major implications for the way in which family responsibilities are seen. We may ask why people feel the obligation to care. This may have to do with love and affection, from the habit of living together, or from other social expectations and values (Arber and Gilbert, 1989). Involving themselves in informal care arrangements requires social workers to be particularly conscious of the social expectations within the family and local community to care and the pressures that this will place on potential carers.

Health and capacity

Health is an important aspect of later life, because older people are more likely than younger people to be ill and to use health services, they are more likely to have several conditions at once, and their reactions may be physically different from younger people (e.g. they feel pain less and drugs affect them differently from younger adults - Swift, 1989, p.137). Much illness relates to environment; there are often causes of illness which derive from environment and life-style. People also become less fit in later life, affecting five aspects of fitness, strength, stamina, suppleness, skill and morale (Tinker et al., 1983). Particular aspects of health, such as nutrition, may become important because financial problems, lack of interest or social isolation (eating is a social activity) may lead to an inadequate intake of necessary foods.

Inevitably, the health status of someone in later life affects their capacity to carry out normal activities of living. So, a higher proportion of older people become disabled by one or other of the degenerative diseases. This may become frustrating and limiting to an older person who has higher expectations, and many fear or dislike the increasingly limited life that disability may force upon them, as did my mother, and envy those that manage to carry on an active existence.

As with many of the factors in later life that we have examined, the response to decline in capacity will vary depending on social expectations around the client and their own wishes and expectations.

Oppression and abuse

We have already noted the possible oppressions of later life which derive from the social position of older people in a society which values youth and emphasises the culture which is associated with young people (Featherstone and Hepworth, 1989). Oppressions deriving from ethnic minority status adds to oppression due to ageism, by leading to the special needs of minority ethnic groups to be ignored (Blakemore, 1989; Fennell et al., 1988, ch.7).

Recent writing has also made us aware of physical abuse (e.g. Eastman, 1984) which may, according to Eastman, include sexual abuse, the misuse of medication, recurring or unexplained injuries, the use of physical constraints, such as tying people to beds or chairs, malnutrition or dehydration and lack of personal care.

In addition, much of the literature on residential care for older people indicates how unsatisfying a life of this kind is for most older people. Sinclair (1988a) summarises the research as showing that most older people do not want to go into residential care, and are not consulted and involved in the move. Booth (1985) found that the outcomes of residential care had nothing to do with how the home was run, but more to do with the life experience, health and personality of older people in care, which gave them the resilience to cope with their experiences in care. Willcocks et al. (1987) in a study of care in local authority homes were struck by how private lives had to be led in a public arena, and recommend that homes should be built and organised to allow residents to gain control over some private territory, and to have individual rights and to take acceptable risks.

A recent study of older people in both community and

residential settings (Allen et al., 1992) emphasises how much satisfaction is increased by older people having choice and active participation in decisions about their affairs. However, present services are very unsatisfactory in this respect. The authors comment (p.312):

> Participation...usually meant acceptance of what was offered - or not offered. Consumer choice, when it was exercised by elderly people, usually took the form of refusing services that were offered, or discontinuing them if they were found unsatisfactory...any participation and choice of the elderly people in the community in the services they received was essentially passive or negative...entering residential care...they simply did not feel themselves up to behaving as active consumers.

Social workers can be aware of many of these oppressions and abuses, in practice both in the community or residential or day care, but providing successful social care for older people must go beyond awareness of the social context that I have emphasised in many of the other aspects of life affecting older people discussed so far. It requires us to implement social care practices in ways which seek to overcome ageism and oppression actively, and support people's capacity to cope with the difficulties they will face in participating in residential care. For example, one project I am currently involved in seeks to strengthen older people's control over a residential setting by making them legally co-owners, employers of the staff, and offering explicit channels for decision-making about their needs individually and collectively.

The question that we must now turn to is how far social work and social care practice is adequate to the task of fostering this kind of participation.

LATER LIFE AND SOCIAL WORK THEORY AND PRACTICE

In discussing the range of social contexts within which social care must be provided, I have tried to show the importance of the social expectations in the community and the experiences and views of older people and their families and social networks. At every point, the social care worker should identify and try to deliver services in accordance with the experience and expectations of an older person which define their own understanding of their needs.

It is in this area of the evaluation and understanding of social experience that the social worker is most skilled and that social work ideas are focused. However, social work theory itself has been underdeveloped in the help it offers to social workers to understand what they are doing with older people, because it largely developed from psychological theories derived from concern about childhood and mental illness, rather than an interest in later life. This is, for example, typical of the psychosocial, behavioural and crisis intervention models of social work which have their origins largely in psychiatric and psychological work (Payne, 1991).

However, other forms of social work theory may be more helpful in working with older people within the social and political contexts that I have argued are so important. An emphasis on communication and cognitive theory, for example, enables us (respectively)

- to gain the skills to understand and work within the communication patterns which reflect the real experience of older people, and
- to acknowledge and accentuate the fact that people can learn about and control their behaviour and environment through their thinking processes rather than being prey to internal emotions and external stresses.

Similarly, ideas like task-centred theory (Reid, 1978) enable us to make more explicit for client involvement and control, the processes through which we seek to intervene in their lives. This is because clear processes for involving the client in defining the problem to be worked on, and participating in a series of identified tasks help to demystify what is going on.

Social care work may also benefit from systems ideas in the form of unitary and integrated theories such as those of Goldstein (1973) and Pincus and Minahan (1973). These theories, although they present theoretical and practical problems (see Payne, 1991), enable social workers to include in their work with individual clients a concept of the linkages with the social networks which may be part of the problem and part of the solution for many clients. More important, these ideas have led on to the development of ideas of networking within social support networks, enabling social workers to concentrate their efforts on developing formal and informal supports for neighbours and family members who are in need (Whittaker and Garbarino, 1983; Walton, 1986; Caplan, 1974).

These ideas suggest how links with support networks can be built up, involving enabling processes, negotiation, mobilising resources within and outside the situation, and advocacy for the client (Payne, 1986; 1993). Eventually, the aim is reciprocity, so that clients can also respond in the network to others' needs, returning some of the resources used to others. Antonucci and Jackson (1989) argue that reciprocity must be seen across the whole lifetime, so that people within older people's networks can feel that they are returning to people in later life the care and support they received from those same people when they were younger. This may involve social workers in identifying and clarifying where older people have been supportive to others in previous years and helping people in the network to respond now to the needs in the people who once helped.

Much of the most helpful of recent writing about social work theory and practice lies in the development of theory about empowerment and advocacy, as developments from radical and Marxist theories of social work. An account of these developments can be found in Payne, M. (1991, chapters 10 and 11). For our purposes, it is important to note how, in advocacy theory as presented by Rose and Black (1985), there is an acceptance that it is not possible to make people independent (and this is true of many people who need social work help in later life) but rather to stimulate interdependence. Rose and Black's (1985) study is of a residential setting, and it is possible to see how residential care practice can be understood in this way. Residential care provides a safe setting with stronger support and help than is usually available in the community to test out risky developments in people's skills. Thus, the interdependence fostered in residential care can stimulate stronger independence for individuals than therapeutic work or services provided in the community.

The crucial new element in these approaches is that they recognise and attempt to work within a political and social understanding of the oppressions faced by clients in a way which involves them and treats them as equals. Thus, in Solomon's (1976) formulation of empowerment theory, the emphasis is specifically on analysis of power or blocks in the use of the client's own power. The aim is to see clients as causal agents who do have the capacity to influence what happens to them, for social workers to work alongside them as partners or as peers in using their knowledge and skills to solve problems and in particular to see the power structure which is actually and potentially oppressive as complex and at least partly open to change for the client's benefit. The work involves identifying power blocks and finding and reinforcing supports to effective problem-solving, and to help clients overcome responses in themselves which cause them to see themselves as unable to act.

Using empowerment with people in later life, the worker would always be seeking ways of using accumulated skills, experience and network reciprocity to give older people at least some room for manoeuvre in affecting their lives. This approach is crucial to meeting the problem identified by Allen et al.'s (1992) research which emphasises the present impossibility of older people becoming realistically involved in making positive choices and taking up active participation in decisions about their lives.

SERVICES AS AN ASPECT OF SOCIAL CARE PRACTICE

Finally, we must turn to the importance within social work with people in later life of the delivery of services. Whereas in work with children and young people and mentally ill people (which is the historical origin of the therapeutic mode of social work and which is the highest status form of social work) direct work with the client is the most prized activity for social workers, much work with people in later life involves the delivery of services. The development of informal networks and empowerment and support needs to be related to the provision of formal, official practical services. Home help, day care, meals, residential care, nursing, occupational therapy and a wide variety of other services have been mentioned throughout this account of social care with people in later life.

Developments in community care in the 1980s and 1990s, while not gainsaying social work practice and theory of the kind discussed in the previous section, has been concentrated on the social services as the manager and provider of a range of services, which need to be better integrated with each other, and provided more effectively with a concern for the interaction of the various costs of service. A report of the Audit Commission on managing social services for older people (Audit Commission, 1985) concentrates on identifying how different local authorities make policy decisions about providing different kinds of services which interact with each other.

Care management, the preferred technique of the Wagner (1988) and Griffiths (1988) Reports, has been integrated into plans for the implementation of the community care aspects of the National Health Service and Community Care Act, 1990 (see for example the official guidance - DoH/SSI/SWSG, 1991). This presumes that at a higher level, the local authority will have planned for a range of care services to be offered. The job of the care manager (perhaps, but not necessarily, a social worker) is to create a package of services individually tailored for each client's needs and including informal and network support, from what is available.

Services, the assessment of their quality and appropriateness and their organisation and management thus become more important. Whereas, at one time, the organisation of service delivery would have been seen as separate from social work tasks, the element of assessment and integration implied in care management as a social care responsibility, bears closely on how services are organised. Recent work by the Department of Health Social Services Inspectorate to identify and make explicit appropriate standards in a number of services (e.g. home care (DoH/SSI, 1990a) and residential care (DoH/SSI, 1989; 1990b) provide detailed statements of the type and manner of provision for services are laid down, based on value principles derived from basic social work ideas. The residential care document (DoH/SSI, 1989) for example, specifically sets out six basic values, privacy, dignity, independence, choice, rights and fulfilment drawn from the social work literature. These values also reflect an attempt to tackle through effective delivery of service, some of the problems identified in the literature discussed above about the dissatisfaction and lack of involvement that older people feel in residential and community care.

We can see here an attempt to integrate into service delivery the importance of understanding about the social context of any social care provision and in so doing to include within the idea of delivery a concept of social care with which I started out in this chapter. That is, social care must be reciprocal and mutual in its form, it must be involving and participative, it must recognise social context and the continuity of life, and it must recognise the reality of the experience of old age, while denying any stereotype of what is 'an elderly person'.

CONCLUSION

If we look at people in later life and their experiences, through the research and practice literature considered here (and much more besides explored in the other chapters in this book) we can move towards a new understanding of how we should view the needs of social care practice and service provision for older people. I have sought to emphasise here how seeing later life as part of a continuity of social experience for each person and social care as a reciprocal and participative process requires us to look at the personal experience and social contexts of each client that workers deal with and the society of which they are a part and how it treats old age. Social work practice must develop advocacy and empowerment strategies alongside conventional individualistic social work practice, it must concern itself with the development of an appropriate community and social context for later life and it must integrate the effective provision of services as part of its central core.

Recent writing about social work practice develops in this direction. Advocacy and empowerment theory, the development of networking and social support strategies and the evolution of care management and attempts at defining and enforcing quality in service provision are all signs of this work going on in the early 1990s. Crucially, this exciting work is directly posited on participation and choice for people in later life in the services and care that they receive, and begins to put social work with older people for the first time in the forefront of the development of social work thinking.

Two:

Aspects of development in later life

Peter Coleman

INTRODUCTION: ATTITUDES TOWARDS AGEING AND DEVELOPMENT

The last 30 years have seen an impressive growth in interest in the study of ageing. Enthusiasm has been kindled across the whole range of academic disciplines, particularly in biology, sociology and psychology but increasingly also in geography, anthropology and economics, and within the humanities as well, especially history. This broadening of interest has led to new questions. We can see better now that the experience of ageing is the product not only of inevitable biological and psychological processes, nor even of the individual's particular life history and present circumstances, but also of the attitudes, expectations, prejudices and ideals of the societies and cultures in which people develop and grow old. Some present day investigators have been led to explore how certain images, models and assumptions about the nature of ageing lie behind everyday speech, and how the very language we use may restrict and inhibit older people, and even promote their decline (Coupland et al., 1991).

It is important therefore to begin this account of current theories and ideas on development in later life with a reflection on the importance of attitudes towards ageing. Not so long ago it would have been thought paradoxical to say the least to include a chapter on 'development' in a book about ageing and care of elderly people. A simplistic picture of the life span as 'rise and fall' is deeply embedded within western culture. It is most graphically depicted in the medieval representations of the 'ages of man', in which the path of later life is one of remorseless decline (Cole, 1992). The idealisation of young adulthood has been attributed by some to an 'iconic triphasic illusion', a gestalt of rise, peak and fall which western culture tends to impose on life experience, as in the familiar domestic mantelpiece with the prized object placed at the top in the centre (Pruyser, 1975). However that may be, it is important to bear in mind that such 'taken for granted' assumptions about the course of life may be very different in other cultures. For example Hindu culture traditionally speaks of stages of life not in terms of rise and fall but of a forward cyclical movement.

Following the period of the Enlightenment, with its emphasis on reason rather than tradition, and the subsequent industrial and technological revolutions, attitudes to older people seem to have become more disrespectful (Fischer, 1978). Their expertise was seen as based on outmoded ways of behaviour and therefore less relevant to a fast changing society. It is not surprising therefore that when the first attempts were made in the 19th century to study scientifically the behaviour and performance of people of different ages, it was natural to adopt a pessimistic stance. Even a thinker as imaginative as Freud conformed to the pattern, viewing people above the age of 40 years as too inflexible to be able to benefit from the practice of psychoanalysis. Such thinking about age is so ingrained in our culture that we are hardly conscious of what we say. It lies behind many of our casual comments about age, such as 'being over the top' and 'past it' and the unflattering depictions of older people in the humour of birthday cards. All such forms of 'ageism', the unjustified attribution of characteristics to persons on the basis of their chronological age, need to be combatted firmly and resolutely and with a skill commensurate to the very considerable forces of prejudice which lie behind them.

The encouragement of positive and constructive attitudes to older people is one of the main themes of this book. We now have the evidence that older people are capable of much more than we sometimes imagine, and that they can be flexible and learn new things. What often holds them back are the negative expectations of others and, perhaps even more importantly, of themselves. But we must also avoid going to the opposite extreme, by almost demanding new qualities from individuals regardless of their circumstances and particular experience of life. As the distinguished French historian of old age Georges Minois (1989) has commented, some of the cruelest societies to the old have been those in which the highest standards of wisdom, serenity and maturity were expected of them. The questions surrounding growth and decline, change and development throughout life are very complex. All one can do in a short commentary as this is select some of the insights from recent studies which throw light on important issues. I shall also consider how this knowledge, provisional though it may be, can be applied in practice.

DIFFERENTIAL AGEING

Above all we need to be discriminating in our approach to older people, sensitive to different needs. The term 'differential' as applied to the study of ageing has become familiar in the last few years. One can identify at least two different senses in which the word is used. The first concerns different domains of functioning. It may be that certain psychological functions deteriorate with age, for example speed of information processing. But others, such as judgements involving important life decisions, may improve, while others still may remain stable. The same point has been made by Neugarten (1988a) in regard to personality. Consistent age differences appear in the inner life, especially intrapsychic processes that are not available to conscious control, for example in the ways persons and events are perceived and in dreams and fantasies. But the outward way in which people respond to events and relate to other people may show little evident change.

The term differential ageing may also be used to refer to differences between types of people in the way that they age. Socio-economic status for example will have a large influence on the life experiences of people after retirement, perhaps even more so than before. This is clear from longitudinal studies of cognition which show that both educational attainment and occupational level influence whether people maintain good intellectual functioning in later life (Schaie, 1990). Studies of personality also show that people react differently to the challenges and stresses that come with age according to their basic orientation to life, their values and coping styles (Neugarten, 1964). Perhaps most important of all as a factor in determining the experience of ageing, its opportunities and general quality of life is the individual's health status. Health is the one element in their life that older people comment on more negatively than younger people.

Further distinctions can also be drawn between the wide range of age groups that make up the older population. Some of these differences may reflect variations between successive generations in their outlook and values. But one broad distinction that is increasingly made reflects the different levels of vitality between what have been called the 'younger old' and 'older old' (Neugarten, 1988b) or more recently the 'third' and 'fourth' ages (Laslett, 1989). One must be careful, though, to define these two groups in terms of health status rather than by chronological age. Although an understandable emphasis is placed on the larger numbers of people who live to a great age within modern societies, the most significant change in fact is the greatly increased number of people who live in good health after retirement. The 'young-old' or 'third-agers' represent a major human resource which is still under-appreciated in most countries.

For those working in the health and social services there is naturally a greater interest in the 'old-old'. Particularly as a result of American studies on elderly people living in institutions (Lieberman and Tobin, 1983), there has been a growing awareness of the distinct psychological features that may characterise the adjustment processes of the very old. The aims of life at this stage may be simpler but also more urgent, to transcend losses by holding to a stable sense of self. In the third age by contrast issues of self-realisation and development may continue to be very important.

We need therefore to recognise the complexity of ageing and apply different considerations to older people according to their circumstances. We also have to strike the right balance and not emphasise the interests of one group of older people to the detriment of the other. Moreover we need to bear in mind that the dichotomous distinction between the 'young-old' and the 'old-old' is itself only a crude one and will need to be replaced by something better when it no longer serves a useful purpose.

In the sections that follow various aspects of development in later life will be considered, beginning with enhanced awareness of death. Death is the key to the psychology of ageing because the sense of its approach brings a changed perspective on life. Most of the major theorists on the psychology of ageing have kept this central truth in mind, and in the subsequent section special attention is given to the work of one of these, the life-span developmental theory of Erik Erikson. This provides important lessons to practitioners about discovering more about the backgrounds of those that they care for, and preserving links with their past lives. One way of doing this is through the encouragement of reminiscence which is the focus of the following section. It is important that all older people are given the opportunity to tell their life story.

The significance of cognitive changes and increased introversion with age are then examined in successive sections. In both cases attention is drawn to the important role of culture and environment in mediating change. The nature of well-being in late life is discussed, including the apparent paradox that older people may at the same time be less happy but more satisfied with their lives than their younger contemporaries. In the penultimate section, particular focus will be given to the challenges posed by physical and mental frailty in advanced old age, and the implications for development at this stage of life. The concluding section provides a brief summary of the main practical points and emphasises again the theme of variation in ageing and the need for an individualised approach.

ACCEPTANCE OF DEATH

It is often said that part of the reason for both the neglect of elderly people in modern western societies and the lack of popularity of work with them is the association of old age with death. Death is a taboo subject in modern western society. As life expectancy has increased so it is predominantly old people who die. As a result the thought of their own death is more easily prevented from entering younger people's awareness. Death is something frequently observed but at the safe distance of the television screen. The close intermingling of life and death, so much part of our ancestors' way of life, leaves most of us uneasy. Only for older people is this a normal state of affairs as friends and acquaintances die in large numbers around them.

The study of ageing itself has often seemed to show scant attention to death. It is as if it too has wanted to avoid contamination. Yet on reflection probably the most profound, and lasting, theoretical contributions to the study of the psychology of ageing are those which have kept death in perspective (e.g. Jung, 1972; Erikson, 1950; Cumming and Henry, 1961; Butler, 1963; Lieberman and Tobin, 1983). In more recent years debates about societal attitudes to death have increased, including the important ethical issues surrounding the subject of euthanasia. Perhaps the gradually improving status of older people in our society is at least in part related to a growing acceptance of discussion about death.

Awareness of death is not only an important matter for those at the end of life, but for all in the 'second part of life' (to use Jung's term). The centrality of death to the psychology of human development in later life was first explicitly addressed in a pioneering study by the Dutch psychologist Joep Munnichs (1966). In a recent formulation of his thinking on the subject of development with age (Munnichs, 1992) he explains how the origins of the changed orientation to life and death usually begin in the middle years, when the reality of the limits on the lifespan make themselves felt. Parents die. Unrealisable aspirations disappear. There is increased introspection, as a result of which both the future and the past come more clearly into focus. The individual's life, as it has been lived so far, comes to be represented as a whole story. Consideration of the future is placed in the context of this developing life history, which while it restricts what is possible also guarantees meaning so long as the link with the past is maintained. The process of personal story and meaning elaboration continues throughout the second part of life, as the life story is made more coherent, clear and memorable.

The attribution of the term 'old' to oneself appears to come with the acceptance of the closeness of death. It is, as Munnichs emphasises, an 'end state' category. To very few genuinely elderly people in fact does death itself appear to be a matter of apprehension, mainly to those few who still feel unfulfilled in their lives (Keith, 1979). The concerns of most elderly people focus rather on the process of dying and the maintenance of the self in the face of death. To have reached this state of mind, of equanimity towards the end of life, is the developmental achievement of old age, but it is something which younger people have difficulty in appreciating.

This formulation of the nature of psychological ageing shows how important it is to try to understand older individuals in terms of their life histories and also to discover how individuals appreciate their own life stories. There has been within personality psychology in recent years a recovery of an interest in studying whole human lives from birth to death and in employing biographical and autobiographical methods to understand persons (McAdams, 1990). Many now acknowledge the pioneering influence of Henry Murray (1938) and of other psychologists who continued to pursue a holistic and life-span approach to studying human lives in opposition to the fashion of the post-war years, which was to analyse particular behaviours and usually only in their immediate context. Of particular significance for the study of ageing have been the writings of Erik Erikson and their emphasis on development over the whole life course.

THE LIFESPAN DEVELOPMENTAL THEORY OF ERIK ERIKSON

Born in Germany Erik Erikson emigrated to the United States in the 1930s as a young adult. Most of his career was devoted to child psychology, in particular in drawing attention to the issues involved in adolescents' search for an acceptable identity. But already in his book 'Childhood and Society' (Erikson, 1950) he went beyond his immediate task by providing a framework for the whole lifespan in terms of a series of tasks to be fulfilled. Thus the child's or rather baby's first psychological task in life is described as developing a sense of trust rather than mistrust. The ensuing childhood stages are characterised in terms of 'autonomy', 'initiative' and 'industry'. In adolescence the issue is the development of 'ego identity' versus 'identity diffusion', perhaps the key stage in his theory, and in early adulthood the development of 'intimacy' versus a sense of 'isolation'.

In middle age the issue becomes one of 'generativity', again a word coined by Erikson. He describes it as 'primarily the interest in establishing and guiding the next generation'. This can mean a focus on one's own family but it can also include broader interests and concerns in the society in which one lives. The opposite state Erikson calls 'stagnation' for which he offers a succinct illustration. 'Individuals who do not develop generativity often begin to indulge themselves as if they were their own one and only child'. The task of the last stage of life, old age, for Erikson is to attain 'ego integrity', an assured sense of meaning and order in one's life and in the universe, as against despair and disgust. This involves 'acceptance of one's one and only life cycle as something that had to be and that, by necessity, permitted of no substitutions' (Erikson, 1965, p.260). Identity is reaffirmed. Despair may be expressed in a feeling that one has failed and does not have the time to attempt another life or an alternative road to integrity, and also in a disgust with other people, especially the young. Erikson's perspective is rooted in his perception of the wholeness of the human life-span: the interdependence of the successive stages of life, the reciprocal relationships between older and younger generations, and the dependence of individual growth upon the social conditions which can foster or also impede development. He expresses this sense of interrelatedness in his poetic comment that 'healthy children will not fear life if their elders have integrity enough not to fear death'.

Erikson's stage model is a radical departure in western thinking, away from the model of rise and decline which became so popular in the middle ages and later (Cole, 1992). It may in fact have more in common with oriental, namely Hindu thinking. Evidence for the validity of a concept such as 'integrity' as applied to old age continues to increase. In studies using self reports, older people rated themselves higher on this dimension (i.e. accepting the limitations of the life cycle and viewing their lives as inevitable, appropriate and meaningful) than they recalled being in the past. Young adults and middle-aged individuals also anticipated scoring higher on 'integrity' in old age than they saw themselves in the present (Ryff and Heincke, 1983). In the most recent reports from the Berkeley longitudinal study in California (Field and Millsap, 1991), which has followed a group of men and women (who were first interviewed in 1928-29 as part of a young parents study) over the period from 'young' (65-74 years) to 'old' (75-84 years) old age, the older people were rated significantly more open-minded, cheerful and accepting. The investigators interpret this in accord with Eriksonian thinking.

It is unfortunate in some ways that discussion of the relevance of Erikson's theory to ageing often focuses on this last stage of 'integrity'. His theory is in fact much more sophisticated than brief presentations often imply. It is not the case that at each stage the 'task' is either left unresolved or resolved, thus allowing the way forward to further development. A solution may be only relatively successful, and this will have repercussions on all subsequent stages. Thus major unresolved residues of earlier difficulties can play a salient part in late life, and make the issues somewhat different for each individual according to his or her own past experience.

Erikson's writings can be illuminating and provide new horizons precisely in those settings where work with older people often seems so dull, as in long-stay hospitals. Archer, for example, provides a telling account of how she came to find added meaning in working with mentally infirm older people on British psychogeriatric wards, through a consideration of each of

Erikson's stages of development (Archer, 1982). It allowed her to recognise each person's individuality, to acknowledge the achievements and struggles different people displayed in maintaining a sense of 'trust' or 'industry' or 'identity', and striving for 'intimacy', 'generativity' and 'integrity'. The insights she gained enabled her to continue responding to the people she cared for as persons and not only as patients.

More recently Helen Kivnick has developed a method for assessing what she describes as 'life strengths' in elderly clients in long-term care which are based on updated versions of Erikson's eight concepts: hope and faith; wilfulness, independence and control; purposefulness, pleasure and imagination; competence and hard work; values and sense of self; love and friendship; care and productivity; wisdom and perspective (Kivnick, 1991). Each of these categories are strengths that the individual older person has built up in unique ways over a long life. When care staff consider residents' or clients' functional needs in isolation from these strengths and values they depersonalise them and exaggerate the relative importance of their disabilities. They unwittingly fail to encourage life-enhancing involvements, and as these are allowed to wither, deficits acquire excessive significance and influence.

THE SIGNIFICANCE OF REMINISCING

One of the many fruits of Erikson's conception of old age as the last but vital part of the life cycle has been a renewed interest in listening to older people reminisce. This is something that even in the 1960s was still frowned on as a result of negative attitudes best encapsulated by Henry Ford's comment that 'history is bunk'. Serious consideration first began to be given to the value of reminiscence in later life after the publication of an article by the American psychiatrist Robert Butler: 'The life review: an interpretation of reminiscence in the aged' (Butler, 1963). Quoting his own clinical experience as well as a wide range of literary authorities, Butler made out a case for viewing reminiscence as a normal activity of old age, and the life review as a process that people may have to undergo if they are to come to terms with their lives. Although in this article Butler made no reference to Erikson, his 'life review' can be considered a means by which a person achieves 'integrity'. Indeed, both Butler (1963) and Erikson (1978) cite Ingmar Bergman's film 'Wild Strawberries', in which an elderly egocentric professor achieves more sensitivity in helping those around him as a result of a process of life review, beginning with disturbing dreams but continuing with conscious recollections of his insensitivity in the past.

Butler's article was followed by a number of other important contributions to the understanding of reminiscence (see Coleman, 1986). Butler had spoken of the 'life review' as a normative and universal process, but others pointed out that elderly people's reminiscence did not always have a searching, enquiring and evaluative character. That phase in their thinking may have long passed. More often older people seemed concerned in their reminiscences to pass on their life story, and to convey the importance and value of their experiences. This reflects the traditional role of the older person as the moral story-teller, and at the same time helps to maintain his or her sense of identity. Such considerations underlie much of current reminiscence work in institutional and community settings. This is not to deny that there is no role for the encouragement of 'life review' itself. Indeed some studies do suggest that it can contribute to a higher level of insight and self-acceptance (Haight, 1988) but, because of the unforeseen difficulties involved in probing a person's secret past life, it should be undertaken responsibly usually in a one to one setting.

It is important to respect the picture an individual has built up of him or herself over a long period, from at least mid-life as Munnichs has indicated. Accuracy is not the only criterion for judging a life narrative. It can also be valued for its coherence, its comprehensiveness and its intelligibility (Cohler, 1982). Understanding how people see their lives is a crucial starting point for deciding the help they will find acceptable. This underlies what is now commonly called the biographical approach to assessment (Gearing and Dant, 1990). However it should perhaps more correctly be called the autobiographical approach, since the focus is on individuals' own understanding of their lives. It has marked advantages over previous approaches to assessment: the worker obtains a more complete picture of the person being assessed; the person's self-esteem is itself enhanced by the skilful encouragement of reminiscence; and links with earlier life are established which often throw light on otherwise puzzling facts about the person's attitudes, family relationships, ways of coping and special needs.

So far, in describing what is common to the psychology of the ageing process, I have not gone further than emphasise a generally increased acceptance of death and the construction of an acceptable life story. I think that these are fundamental to our present understanding of the developmental tasks of later life and, as Erikson shows, provide important lessons for those who follow after. But there may be other developmental features too, such as an enhanced capacity for wisdom and for spiritual growth, which also have social as well as individual value.

WISDOM AND THE DEVELOPMENT OF NEW ABILITIES

Unfortunately much of the early work on the psychology of ageing focused on intelligence and especially the now less accepted notion of 'general intelligence' (IQ). Studies purported to chart the negative changes through later life, but neglected the more important influences due to education (Coleman, 1994). Recent longitudinal studies show that the basic mechanisms of intelligence remain relatively stable until the influences of poorer health and biological ageing make themselves felt in late life. More relevant to behaviour throughout the second half of life are the particular kinds of intelligence or repertoires of ability that the individual continues to develop. Such abilities are essentially pragmatic, related to the way an individual copes with his or her own particular situation in life, and can only be appropriately studied in the natural settings in which they occur.

Intelligence tests in fact become more inadequate the longer people have lived and have acquired, as a result, different experiences from one another (Dittmann-Kohli and Baltes, 1990). Such tests may be capable of measuring age decline but not age improvement. They do not do justice to the complex and socially valued activities that many people develop over a long lifetime. To assess such developments one would need tests attuned to the specialist activities of the people in question, whether politicians, writers, managers or therapists. There is considerable variation in the knowledge and problem-solving skills required for the different positions in life people hold, and they consequently come to vary considerably in the domains of expertise they possess. This expertise can be heightened by further challenges. It can decline through lack of use, but it remains as essential a part of people's adjustment to their life situation as the basic 'fluid' intelligence potential they were born with.

While expertise can distinguish people, it can also limit them. Indeed some of the problems of old age may relate to overspecialisation, and inability to pursue new ways of thinking, feeling and behaviour which are required by new circumstances.

Nevertheless, some people as they age succeed in acquiring a greater general expertise in dealing with the problems life sets. This is a good approximate definition to 'wisdom', which we recognise as a generalised form of intelligence in judging life situations that are both important and uncertain. Attempts to study wisdom empirically are very recent and have begun by delineating the key characteristics of wise judgements, and developing suitable means to assess them. However it is already clear that older people are over-represented among those who display 'wise' judgements when asked to respond to problematic life situations (Baltes et al., 1992).

It is vitally important for all societies to cultivate wisdom in their older people. It is interesting to consider whether we in our professional lives, for example those working in residential homes, would consider asking advice from the elderly people we care for, and if not why not? As Erikson and Kivnick have stressed (Kivnick, 1991) older people need to be given opportunities to reciprocate care and concern, and contribute from their own store of life experience, for all our benefit.

Some of the most interesting studies on older people's learning are those that focus on real-life situations. For example, Harwood and Naylor in Australia (Naylor and Harwood, 1975) investigated a group of 80 volunteers aged 63 to 91 years in an exercise in which they were expected to learn German from scratch - a convenient choice for a naturalistic study of learning since learning to read a foreign language is not difficult to assess quantitatively. The learners were remarkably successful. After six months the majority of people had reached a level of skill in reading German which normally takes schoolchildren five years to achieve. A study by the same group on the learning of recorder playing was likewise very successful.

These volunteers had the 'flexibility' of mind which appears to be an important asset in the process of ageing. The point is not that we should expect all older people to want to learn a foreign language or to play a musical instrument. Rather it is that older people should be more likely to know what are the activities for which they do have the skills and inclination, and also to know better their weaker points. In their recent in-depth consideration of what is involved in 'successful ageing' Paul and Margaret Baltes emphasise the principles of 'selection' (concentrating on those activities that are of high priority and suit one's skills and situation), 'optimisation' (making sure one gets right what is realiy important), and 'compensation' (making adaptations that minimise the impact of weaknesses) (Baltes and Baltes, 1990). They cite an interview with the pianist Arthur Rubinstein, which provides an apt illustration of the principles in question. His own account of the ways in which he overcame his weaknesses with age in piano playing included playing a smaller number of pieces (selection); practising these more often (optimisation); and slowing down his speed of playing before fast movements, thereby producing a contrast that enhanced the impression of speed in the fast movements (compensation).

Musicians and artist have advantages over their contemporaries in modern society in that they continue to receive encouragement to work and be creative as they grow older. The role of social attitudes in older people's cognitive decline is as yet a little explored subject, but will become more recognised as older people themselves begin to resist social stigmatisation, as has already happened in the United States. The most telling empirical studies so far have been experiments in American homes for elderly people where attempts have been made to reverse the spiral of decline. Competent behaviour is often undermined by the attitudes and practices of staff working within institutions. Even minor interventions can change the situation dramatically, for instance giving people more control over what is happening to them and involving them more (Rodin, 1986). Improvements in mental alertness and increased involvement in activities as well as high adjustment levels have been reported from controlled studies where residents have been encouraged to take the initiative for themselves (Langer, 1989). This is not an easy matter when people have long been used to having decisions made for them, but it is possible.

INCREASED INTERIORISATION

Although some longitudinal studies of personality traits indicate considerable stability with ageing (McCrae and Costa, 1990), many studies do indicate a steady shift on the introversion-extraversion dimension towards introversion. This also appears to be the case from 'young' to 'old' old age according to the already mentioned Berkeley longitudinal study (Field and Millsap, 1991). Although relatively easy to demonstrate, this finding is less easy to explain. It is important to appreciate what 'turning inwards' can mean. One of the common stereotypes about older people is that they are 'self-centred'. This is often given a negative connotation by observers including care workers, but may reflect a youthful perspective in a society as ours which also tends to favour extraverts. Jung was one of the first psychologists to comment on and look positively at growing interiorisation with age. It was also observed in the first major cross-sectional study on personality change with age in the USA which gave rise to the so-called 'disengagement theory' (Cumming and Henry, 1961). The authors argued that ageing represented an inherent and universal process of mutual withdrawal between the individual and society. From their perspective the successful agers were the persons who had disengaged and who also welcomed the resulting greater social distance and decreased social interaction.

It is important to bear in mind that the original theory of disengagement was set up consciously as a reaction to what the authors regarded as the underlying 'theory' of ageing current in American society at the time, namely that ageing is intrinsically deteriorative and that 'successful ageing consists in being as much like a middle-aged person as possible'. Cumming and Henry challenged this view but probably went too far in their defence of social withdrawal. The issue has continuing important implications for practice. Should care services be organised so as to keep older people stimulated and engaged, or should people be allowed to sit and think if that appears to be their wish? The answer seems to lie in a more sensitive appreciation of individual needs. In a pioneering study of personality and adaptation Neugarten showed how 'certain personality types seem to slough off various role responsibilities with relative comfort and to remain highly content with life' whereas 'for others who show a drop in social interaction there is a drop in life satisfaction' (Neugarten, 1988).

The concept of disengagement has been placed in a larger context by studies of ageing in other cultures. On the basis of research in a variety of traditional societies around the world, in which he often succeeded in tracing and interviewing the same individuals after a time lapse of many years, Gutmann arrives at some provocative conclusions (Gutmann, 1987). He argues that in modern western society we both miss the evident strengths that older people do display, such as the capacity to adjust to loss, and at the same time do not allow them to exploit their full potential. Development is easier to observe in more traditional societies because these societies provide the necessary circumstances for older people to flourish, namely a coherent culture with well defined traditions. In his thinking on this point Gutmann shows the influence of studying under Erikson. Just as a maternal figure is vital to development in infancy, and a peer group is crucial to the formation of identity in adolescence, so a well-rooted culture appears to be a necessary requirement for later life to achieve its real potential.

In traditional societies, Gutmann claims, older people come to take on new roles as 'emeritus parents' - thus echoing Erikson's developmental task of 'generativity'. While women become more assertive and powerful within the realm of the extended family, older men do indeed appear to 'disengage' from the world of pragmatic action, but in order to become tenders of the values of their cultures. Their detachment from ordinary affairs frees them to make this advance so that they represent the abstract but vital elements underlying their culture. They do this by engaging closely in the moral values and religious practices which underlie their cultures. In doing so they gain new meaning in their own eyes and in the eyes of others.

Gutmann had worked as a younger researcher on the earlier 'disengagement' study, but as a result of his comparative studies has come to see the disengagement of older people observed in the United States to be the result of loss of natural roles in society. Both older men and women have lost their vital function in renewing and strengthening the basis of their culture. The recovery of the role of elders and the recovery of culture, Gutmann claims, go hand in hand. Indeed some of the saddest studies on ageing are those which depict older people who cannot come to terms with cultural and moral change in the world around them, sometimes as a result of physical relocation from their culture of origin, but more likely as a result of spiritual isolation from their own society (Francis, 1984; Coleman and McCulloch, 1990).

An important point that emerges from Gutmann's work is that increased interiorisation with age does not have to mean disengagement. As they become older it may be that people become more rooted in their inner selves, and derive both energy and sense of direction from inside. But at the same time they may have much more to give to others from their consolidated experience and from the present example of their lives. It is vital for the health of society, both Erikson and Gutmann claim, for older people to continue to contribute and not to isolate themselves from the rest of society. There is a danger that we may be creating a society where experience between generations will become incommunicable (Moody, 1984).

WELL-BEING IN LATER LIFE

It was mentioned earlier that one reason for viewing old age negatively is its close association with death in our society. But another is the number of losses and difficulties, which older people face more frequently than their younger counterparts. Bereavements occur more often, and declining health deprives people of fitness, and favourite activities, pastimes and roles. Sometimes people comment that it must be terrible to grow old! Yet the numbers of people who become clinically depressed in late life are low, certainly much lower than one would expect on the basis of studies which have demonstrated close links between life stresses and depression in younger adults. It does appear that as people age they acquire certain compensating strengths, as Gutmann suggests.

Further convincing evidence for a growing adaptive capacity is the fact that numerous studies show, contrary to expectation, that self-esteem remains high in late life (Baltes and Baltes, 1990). In studies which have explored changing self-perceptions with age by means of sentence-completion questionnaires (e.g. 'when I think about myself I ......'), systematic differences have been found between young adults and older people (Dittmann-Kohli, 1990). The past is an important aspect of the latter's identity but not the former's. There is also a qualitative change in future perspective: young adults look to the future for roles, hopes and dreams where they will realise themselves, whereas for older adults the future is where, if all goes well, present positive conditions can be maintained. It is older people who are more positive about their present lives and selves, while the young are more self-critical.

The extent and quality of these changes suggest that they are genuine developmental changes rather than generational differences. A new meaning system has been developed for interpreting the changing experiences of life. Similar observations have been made by Heim (1990). She reports that she had initially not considered asking her respondents about the positive aspects of growing old in her investigation, but when she did was surprised at how many positive features were recounted. A number commented on becoming more self-accepting, becoming more tolerant and less irritable, having a heightened sensation for and more appreciation of natural beauty (flowers, sunsets, landscapes), feeling strong emotions less intensely, and an understanding that things matter less.

Whereas many elderly persons report some depressive symptoms, such as loneliness and low moods, there is no more clinical depression among elderly persons than among persons of younger ages (Henderson, 1989). In studies which have investigated the relationship between different dimensions of life satisfaction and age, mood did show some decline with age but was balanced by other factors such as increased self-esteem and congruence between desired and achieved goals (Neugarten et al., 1961; Campbell et al., 1976). In other words there appears to be a shift from 'happiness' to 'satisfaction'. Disappointments become acknowledged as part of life. Losses are accepted without overmuch preoccupation. We notice those elderly people who do become depressed, but pay less attention to the far greater number who withstand loss well, perhaps because they are harder to identify with. Yet theirs is the more typical achievement of late life, an acceptance of life as it is and as it has been lived. Our ability to make sense of things and to find meaning in life does not decline with age. In fact as studies on age difference in cognition seem to indicate, older people become more skilled in the creation and transmission of meaning.

THE PSYCHOLOGY OF LATE LIFE

I have depicted normal psychosocial ageing as a positive process towards greater acceptance of self, life and society and towards becoming a role model for others. An older person does not have to be a paragon of virtue to provide the important sign that life is meaningful and has worth and value. The end result is well captured in Erikson's term 'integrity'. But what happens after this process has reached completion or is threatened by the devastating losses of late life? Not everyone lives to be dependent and frail but increasing numbers do. Do the issues change? Erikson himself has considered this question. In the ninth decade of his own life he designed a follow-up study to the Berkeley longitudinal study (Erikson et al., 1986), in which he discussed the challenges to older people's state of integrity posed by modern society. He stressed the importance of continued 'involvement'.Other theorists, notably Tobin (1991), have argued that the psychology of the very old and frail is indeed different. This has long been recognised by researchers in the concept of 'terminal drop', in which cognitive deterioration precedes death, but there appear to be other distinct features as well.

When people reach this stage of life, they are prepared even in our ageist society to accept the attribution 'old' of themselves. Munnichs (1992) emphasises that perceiving oneself as old is synonymous with accepting the closeness of death. Concern with death itself is likely to have disappeared. There is more concern with the process of dying, particularly dying alone or in pain. All people, old as well as young, wish to keep in control of their lives right to the end. We also wish to remain ourselves in the face of death, not to turn into someone or something we would not recognise as ourselves.

A number of detailed studies carried out by Lieberman and Tobin (1983) have examined how elderly people in the United States adapt to the stress of relocation to institutional care. In interpreting their findings it is important to bear in mind the trauma involved in institutionalisation in a society which prizes independent living even more than its British counterparts. The studies demonstrate the remarkable stability of self image that people maintain across these transitions, but this is often achieved by changing the basis on which the self is constructed. Rather than relying on incidents from their current interpersonal interactions to confirm their image of self, people in these situations of loss and transition also give many examples from their past lives as well as general statements of conviction. They even seem prepared to forego present reality altogether and use evidence based on wishes and distortions to maintain self-consistency.

Such behaviour can seem disturbing at first acquaintance, as when an elderly resident refers to a picture taken 50 years ago as if it was a picture of her today. But this illustration serves to emphasise what has been said already about the achievement of a coherent life story in late life. To an older person, identities are persistent. She or he is not the frail, impaired person you see but the sum - an integrated sum - of a long series of life experiences and events, of which the last may be of relatively little importance.

Other features noted in the psychology of the very old by these researchers include a mythicising of the past, a dramatisation in which the important people and events become 'bigger and better'. The greater vividness, the recall of feelings of love and devotion from parents and others, create a sense of specialness. Kaufman (1987) has also illustrated how older persons transform present experience in ways that conform to important themes of their lives. It is the theme, for example of being the loved mother of a united family, that provides the persistent sense of meaning even when the reality fails to match.

In other ways though, very old people may show a truer awareness, particularly of their own feelings. Destructive and anti-social feelings are admitted without the embarrassment and defensive explanations that might have been elicited earlier in life. According to Tobin (1991) this is because even previously unwelcome motives can be useful for self-definition in the face of the losses of old age. They affirm who one is and has been. Coherence and wholeness can be and are achieved, Tobin argues, even by those 'whose reminiscence is unfortunately filled with vivid and (most likely) accurate memories of losses and deprivation'. These same American studies of relocation to institutions show that it is the elderly people who are prepared to be more assertive and combative in defining their own interests who survive longer. Passivity - including accepting how others define one - leads to earlier decline. Whether these findings hold true of British institutions remains to be seen. Whatever the outcome Lieberman and Tobin deserve our thanks for raising the issue of the adaptive psychology of the very old.

In advanced old age therefore the practical implications may be less to do with fostering psychological development than supporting people in their efforts to stay as they are. One way to do this is, as already noted, through encouraging reminiscence. Personal possessions which provide a tangible link with past activities are very important as well. Religious and cultural practices also offer a valuable source of continuity with previous life for those who have found them meaningful before. American studies also demonstrate the particular significance of religious cognitions in coping with stress in later life (Koenig, 1992). British elderly people are perhaps less religious than their American counterparts, but the provision of opportunities for contact with religious traditions needs to be given greater emphasis in both residential and domiciliary care provision for elderly people.

SUMMARY: LESSONS FOR PRACTICE

A major emphasis in this chapter has been on the importance of a differential approach to ageing and to the experience of people at different stages and in different circumstances within the life course. We need to become more responsive to individuals' real needs and not be misled by stereotyped thinking about what is good for 'all old people'. Stages can be observed within the ageing process. For example the frail elderly person's needs for support and understanding are quite distinct from the fit and healthy 'younger' person's needs to make a continuing contribution. But the fact of a general association with age should not prevent us from acknowledging and responding appropriately to the vitality of many people in their 80s and even 90s. Furthermore, just because a person may have 'fourth age' needs in some respects, by being wheelchair bound for example, it does not follow that he or she should not also partake in 'third age' living. Appropriate use of transport and/or information technology would be sufficient to enable participation in a U3A ('University of the Third Age') or other educational class.

We can find out much about people's needs by learning about their backgrounds. Old age is the product of a long life and needs to be understood in that context. Erikson's concepts have been found useful because they refer to a person's characteristics, like their capacity for 'trust', for 'intimacy' and for 'generativity', which have been shaped over a life-span and continue to seek a positive resolution before death. Attempts, as Kivnick's, to construct an assessment schedule for use in long term care settings to assess older people's 'strengths' are much needed. They help place 'deficiencies' in their proper context. Such assessment should start from people's own view of themselves and their lives. One way of approaching a sensitive decision about care (eg whether to enter a home or not) is to explore with the person the life story so far and to see what would fit best as the next chapter.

It is important to preserve links between an older person's past and present. Sometimes in the turmoil of a move to a residential home, possessions that could have helped preserve a sense of identity are left behind. Encouragement of reminiscence can also promote a sense of a life that has been lived well, despite the setbacks and missed opportunities. In extreme old age it appears that people need, sometimes desperately, to hang on to a sense of who they have been. Care workers should be sympathetic and tolerant to the more extreme manifestations of this need for stability of self, as in repetitions of self defining life stories, exaggerations and the creation of 'myths'. This search for security may be more pronounced in a fast changing society as ours with weaker cultural roots. Celebration of traditional festivals and religious services have an important part to play in preserving a sense of continuity for those to whom they have been significant parts of their lives.

Although the provision of opportunities for reminiscence has important intrinsic value for the person in helping to relive past times and to reassess significant and traumatic events, its greatest value is when it allows the older person to perform the traditional role of story teller and pass on important messages to a younger generation. We should seek out opportunities for older people to continue giving from their accumulated wisdom and experience, including the ways in which they have dealt with major losses. Our society does not always offer them enough challenges to maintain their expertise, to be mindful of what is happening around them, and to give practical help and advice. We let older people disengage and both older and younger generations suffer as a result.

I began this chapter by emphasising how societal attitudes and the very language we use shape older people's lives for better and worse. In harming older people's prospects we also do damage to our own identity of course, by failing to respect our origins and by casting a shadow over our future destination. If older people have no special place or purpose ultimately we too have nowhere to go. Just as the different parts of the life course are interconnected so too are the fates of the different generations. Those in the caring professions are given a special responsibility to help people construct a meaningful and satisfying end to their life story. Seen in its true light this is quite awesome. It has yet to be fully recognised.

Three:

Later life in a social context

John Bond

INTRODUCTION

This chapter will explore the social context of later life. It examines the way that later life is constrained by images and stereotypes of ageing and the way that negative attitudes reinforce ageism in British society. One feature of later life, which helps to create negative stereotypes, is the belief that ill-health and disability are synonymous with old age. We shall see that although ill-health and disability are features of the ageing experience, that healthy living in later life is increasingly common nowadays. The resources of individuals in later life will be examined and we will reflect on the negative and positive aspects of ageing within the context of social relations.

The social construction of later life

Sociologists study human ageing from a variety of perspectives. One approach has highlighted the way that societies construct social facts. For example, biological models have played a central role in explaining the ageing process. A number of biological theories of ageing have been developed from the simple observation that most living organisms show an age-related decline in functional performance (Bond et al., 1993). A number of the criteria delineated by Strehler (1962) have been widely accepted:

- ageing is *universal*, in that it occurs in all members of the population;

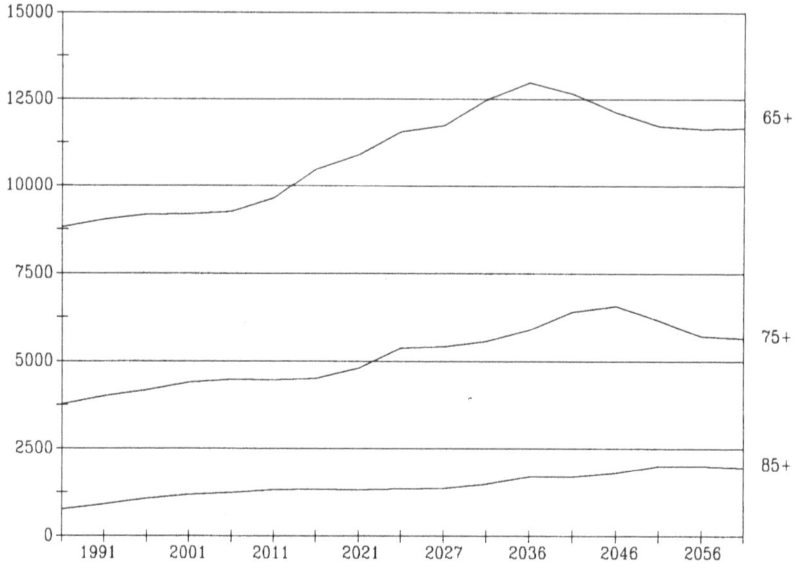

Figure 3.1 *Projected population of elderly people (in thousands) in the United Kingdom 1987–2057*

Source: Population Projections 1989–based. Series PP2 No 17. London: HMSO

- ageing is *progressive*, a continuous process;
- ageing is *intrinsic* to the organism, and therefore inevitable;
- ageing is *degenerative*.

Although ageing and death are inevitable features of human life, biological theories help explain the wide variation in the course of individuals' ageing trajectories. Sociologists have highlighted the way in which the biological perspective has been used to explain social ageing. Society has constructed the social category of old age using biological data to support the view that all individuals follow a similar trajectory from birth to death. Thus chronological age determines transition from childhood to adulthood and from economically active to economically inactive. Such structural features of our society help sustain and underpin common stereotypes about human ageing. The corruption of the biological model in this way ignores the important observation that ageing is unique to individual organisms, including human organisms. Thus in everyday life you will have all met the athletic octogenarian competing in a marathon, as well as the frail octogenarian housebound by debilitating chronic disease. Yet it will be the latter experience that is used to reinforce your own attitudes and stereotypes.

Table 3.1: Images of later life

- Wise and passive elderly people who do not take part in life but who present themselves as moral and affable members of society
- Elderly people who do not conform to the above stereotype and who refuse to adopt the roles of later life prescribed by society
- Men and women who are very frail. Often described as 'senile' or 'geriatric' in everyday life.

Demographic stereotypes

A preoccupation among planners and politicians in the latter part of the twentieth century has been the observation that the absolute number of older people is increasing while the number of individuals in younger age groups is declining. Old age is seen as a problem or a burden. It is not surprising that so many of our elderly citizens should feel that they are a burden. This is not to deny the challenge to society of the demographic changes shown in Figure 3.1 or the poor quality of life experienced by many elderly people. It is, however, disappointing that the joys and triumphs of later life have not been so energetically proclaimed. The view that sees the rising numbers of elderly people as a disaster or problem should be combated with vigour, otherwise it will be a self-fulfilling prophesy (Coleman et al., 1993).

ATTITUDES TOWARDS PEOPLE IN LATER LIFE

In their introduction to social gerontology, Coleman et al. (1993) emphasise the importance of social attitudes towards elderly people as the key to understanding the social context of later life. The biological model of ageing has been used to justify common perceptions of later life: disability, senility, powerlessness and loneliness. A historical view highlights that negative attitudes towards later life are not only a feature of the twentieth century (Featherstone and Hepworth, 1993). A study of the period dating from 1300-1840 by MacFarlane (1986) illustrates how individuals with diminished physical, financial and social resources were often neglected and despised. An analysis of art and literature during the Victorian era led Featherstone and Hepworth (1993) to identify a three-fold distinction between the 'good old', the 'bad old' and those simply 'past it' (see Table 3.1).

Thus the images of later life in pre-industrial and industrial society did not suggest a tradition of interest in growing old or an optimistic prospect for later life. They do, however, highlight the diversity of images held about later life and the discrepancy between our own experiences of individual elderly people and society's enduring stereotypes.

Our changing images of elderly people in the twentieth century although securely locked into history have been particularly influenced by modernity and the value systems of a modern consumer culture. We emphasise youthfulness and the energy of youth. The processes of modernisation and technological innovation render the skills and knowledge of older generations redundant. As a society we invest in youth, 'our future', rather than in the retraining and education of people in later life. Older workers are encouraged to take early retirement rather than investing in their retraining. As a result of this increased social change, we have all become increasingly age conscious. The stereotypical age categories handed down from pre-industrial and industrial society have been expanded by experts such as medical scientists, economists and management consultants, among others, to underpin the age-stratified society and reinforce ageism.

Overcoming ageism

In most European countries people who are economically inactive are devalued and considered irrelevant to the production process. They are perceived as a burden since they are not part of the modern economy. Yet they remain an important part of the social economy. Not just as consumers, in which people in later life play a major part, but as providers of social goods such as historical knowledge or companionship.

Ageism, the negative stereotyping of individuals on the basis of age, is institutionalised in the UK and other European societies. Elderly people are denied certain citizenship rights and have limited access to social, political and economic power. Ageist attitudes are expressed in the behaviour of personal social services and health service staff who treat patients and clients as dependent children through invoking cultural metaphors of childhood (Hazan, 1980; Hockey and James, 1990). Practices such as infantilisation at one level may be regarded as being an unfortunate but inevitable response to human dependency. On another level, however, the metaphoric strategies of ageism can be seen as one means of creating and maintaining the powerful social categories between them, the aged and infirm, and us the younger and abler members of society.

Without political will and sustained social pressure it will be extremely difficult to eradicate institutionalised ageism. We will need more than just statutory legislation like the Race Relations Act before overcoming the effects of ageism. Importantly society will need to provide more resources in the form of increased pensions, better access to high quality housing and increased community and residential services. With competition from other public services for scarce resources the likelihood of making an impact on ageism at the macro level seems remote.

At the micro level, however, there are opportunities to have a substantial impact on ageism. Through education and example professionals and other care workers could change their attitudes and approach to elderly people. But as we have seen this change would not come about overnight and would need the sustained effort of all those on a day to day basis in our interactions with clients. Managers should take the lead in formal organisations and identify a target to rid the organisation of all features of ageism. A lot can be done without the use of financial resources.

HEALTH AND ILL-HEALTH IN LATER LIFE

As we have seen many of the negative attitudes which society has about later life are rooted in the effects of illhealth and infirmity. Numerous epidemiological surveys, surveys undertaken to estimate the prevalence of disease or disability, show an increased prevalence with chronological age. Blaxter (1990) reports data from a survey of some 9000 adult respondents on health and lifestyle. Figure 3.2 (see p.48)shows the marked relationship between chronological age and three indices of health used by Blaxter: a level of fitness based on physiological measures ('fitness/unfitness'); presence of disease and impairment based on reported medically-defined conditions and the degrees of disability which accompany them ('disease/ disability'); and presence of illness based on reports of symptoms suffered ('illness'). The figure uses 'standardised health ratios' to show the relative health experience of men and women in different age groups. The 'standardised health ratio' for each of the three dimensions of health shown represents the relationship of a group to the mean value on each scale found in the population. A value of 100 represents the mean. A lower value represents

Figure 3.2 **Health rates for three dimensions of health by age and gender (total population mean = 100)**

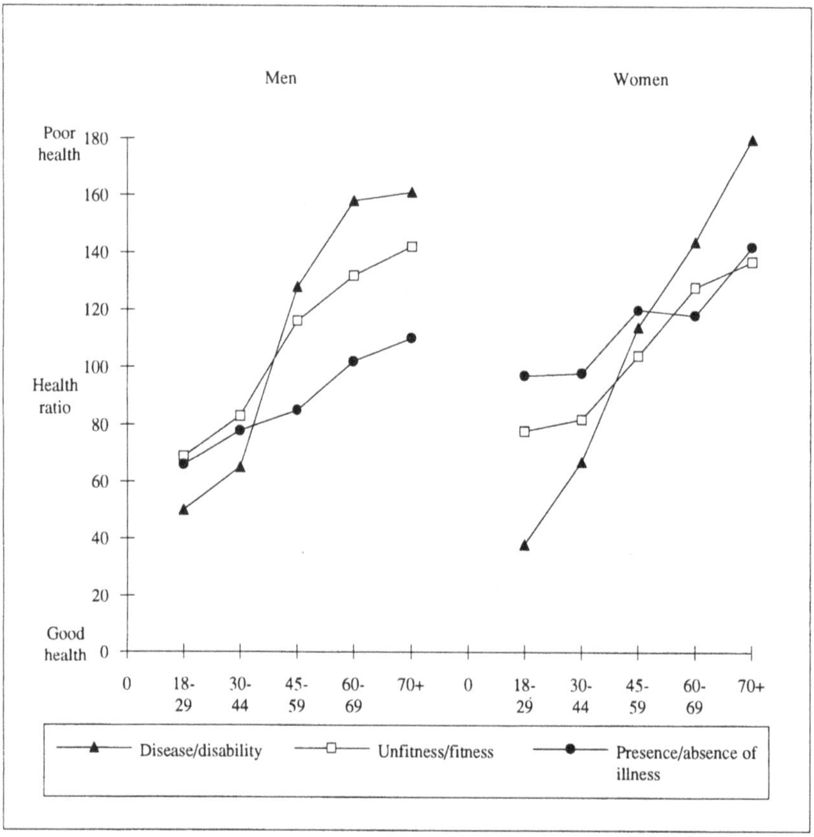

Source: Blaxter, M. (1990) *Health and Lifestyles* London: Tavistock/Routledge. Figure 4.1

less illhealth than the mean. For example, a value of 70 on the 'fitness/unfitness' scale means that this group are 30% fitter than the average. Conversely, a higher value represents more illhealth than the mean. Thus, a value of 130 on the 'fitness/unfitness' scale means that this group are 30% less fit than the average. For each dimension shown, the lower the figure, the better the relative health.

Such data, which underpin ageism, also fuel our own personal fears about later life. They do, however, mask the enormous variability in the prevalence of disability and infirmity at each age year of life.

Health problems of later life

In later life we are more likely to experience both acute and chronic health problems than when we were younger (Victor, 1991). What kinds of health problems are the experience of people in later life? We can use data from the General Household Surveys of 1980 and 1985, prepared by the Office of Population Censuses and Surveys (OPCS, 1982; 1988), the health and lifestyle survey (Blaxter, 1990), the national disability survey (Martin et al., 1988) and numerous psychiatric epidemiological surveys to highlight the health problems of later life.

ACUTE HEALTH PROBLEMS

Acute health problems are self-limiting conditions of short duration such as colds or 'flu or conditions which have a clear recovery trajectory such as fractures of the leg or arm. Data from the General Household Survey (GHS) on restricted activity provides a general indication of the extent of acute illness in a population. In the GHS respondents are asked whether in the 14 days prior to the interview they have had to cut down on normal activities because of illness or injury. Those who report restricted activities are asked to say for how many days they were restricted. The self-reported prevalence of acute health problems based on restricted activity is quite low among elderly people, although higher than the rest of the population. Elderly women reported more restricted activity than men (see Table 3.2, p.50).

Another way at looking at acute health problems is to consider common symptoms reported by elderly people. Using data from the Health and Lifestyles Survey we can see that for some symptoms there are marked gender differences (Table 3.2). For example, whereas the reported prevalence of colds and 'flu in the last month is similar for men and women, about a quarter reporting such symptoms, women were more likely to report painful joints, trouble with eyes, trouble with feet and headaches than men. Differences in the way that men and women report certain symptoms may account for the higher prevalence rates among women (Miles, 1991).

CHRONIC HEALTH PROBLEMS AND DISABILITY

In later life the inevitable consequences of physiological decline sooner or later catch up with us. Unlike the universal nature of this decline, which we have noted operates differentially between individuals, disease is sporadic, only affecting certain members of the population. In later life, however, there is a higher risk of

Table 3.2: Acute health problems in later life

	65-74		75 or over	
	Men	Women	Men	Women
	%	%	%	%
Restricted activity[1]	14	20	18	23
Common symptoms				
Painful joints	28	43	35	48
'Bad back'	17	28	25	31
Breathlessness	22	28	27	31
Trouble with eyes	15	27	25	38
Trouble with ears	21	17	23	22
Trouble with feet	16	23	23	38
Indigestion	21	23	18	23
Headache	13	25	23	21
Cold/flu	26	27	27	23

Sources:

1. *Office of Population Censuses and Surveys (1988)* General Household Survey 1985. *London: HMSO. Table 4.1.*
2. *Blaxter, M. (1990)* Health and Lifestyles. *London: Routledge and Kegan Paul. Table 4.3.*
   Cox, B,D., Blaxter, M., Buckle, A,L,J. et al. (1987) The Health and Lifestyle Survey: Preliminary Report. *London: The Health Promotion Research Trust. Table 2.6.*

disease and many diseases such as stroke or Alzheimer's disease are age related. One of the problems in estimating the prevalence of chronic health problems in later life is co-morbidity, where a combination of diseases are confounded by physiological decline. In addition to the multiple disabilities caused by the diseases themselves, complications may arise due to the complexity of pharmacological interventions. A further problem in identifying the relevance of disease in later life is one of severity. A single diagnosis may affect individuals in different ways ranging from a minor irritation to profound health and lifestyle consequences.

In population studies it has therefore been found more useful to measure the effect chronic health problems have on the individual rather than the prevalence of specific diseases. In the GHS chronic health problems are identified through questions concerned with long-standing illness, disability or infirmity and whether reported conditions limit activities in any way

Table 3.3: Chronic health problems

	65-74		75 or over	
	Men	Women	Men	Women
	%	%	%	%
Longstanding illness	60	63	69	73
Longstanding Limiting illness	43	45	56	58

***Sources**: Office of Population Censuses and Surveys (1988)* General Household Survey 1985. *London: HMSO. Table 4.1.*

(Table 3.3). As with acute health problems elderly women are more likely than elderly men to report long-standing illness or long-standing limiting illness.

Disability can be assessed by a variety of methods. The simplest and most durable has been through the measurement of functional disability based on individuals' abilities to undertake activities of daily living. This has been particularly successful in population studies where self-reported data are collected. The OPCS disability survey, however, uses the International Classification of Impairments, Disabilities and Handicaps as the basis for defining people with disabilities in ten main areas (Martin et al., 1988). Estimates of the prevalence of each type of disability is shown in Table 3.4 (see p.52).

MENTAL HEALTH PROBLEMS IN LATER LIFE

One of the fears of politicians and the government is the increasing dependency of elderly people on the State caused by mental health problems particularly the group of diseases of organic origin classified as dementia. The prevalence of dementia is reported as about 5% for people aged 65 years or over and up to 20% for those aged 80 years or over. It is estimated the prevalence doubles every seven years (Jorm, 1990).

Elderly people also suffer from depression and other functional psychiatric illnesses for which there exists no identified organic cause. It is the commonest psychiatric illness of later life identified in epidemiological surveys. Depression is probably the epidemic condition of later life. Prevalence estimates are notoriously unreliable, however, ranging from 6 to 26% in recent British studies (Brayne and Ames, 1988).

It is essential, however, to emphasise that the majority of people in later life remain as independent of help from others as

Table 3.4: Types of disability

	60 - 74	75 and over
	%	%
Locomotion	20	50
Reaching and stretching	5	15
Dexterity	8	20
Seeing	6	26
Hearing	11	33
Personal care	10	31
Continence	4	15
Communication	4	14
Behaviour	4	15
Intellectual functioning	4	11

***Source**: Martin, J., Meltzer, H. and Elliot, D. (1988) Office of Population Censuses and Surveys* Disability Surveys, Report 1: The Prevalence of Disability Among Adults. *London: HMSO. Table 3.14.*

do younger people. Stereotypes of elderly people as confused, depressed and chronically infirm are unwarranted. There are only a minority of sufferers who may require extensive support at any one time. When they do need this support, it can be considerable.

LIVING ARRANGEMENTS IN LATER LIFE

One of the most influential factors on all our lives is the environment in which we live. This may be increasingly so in later life since we are more likely to spend time in our own homes. The physical location of the homes of elderly people will influence their continuing health as well as their ability to cope with illhealth and disability. If, as we get older, we live a long way from food shops, at the top of a steep hill or in a busy urban area we may find it difficult to remain independent and increasingly rely on other people to get our shopping and to take us out.

An increasing trend of recent years has been the migration of people around retirement age away from the areas in which they have lived during their working lives. Retirement migration, however, is still a minority activity which affects about ten per cent of the elderly population (Law and Warnes, 1982). It is most likely to be the experience of seasoned migrants who have moved relatively frequently in their working lives and of those who are relatively affluent. Most people do not wish to move or are unable to do so. Elderly migrants create a particular challenge in those areas of the country known as the 'costa geriatrica' since incoming migrants have frequently no established social networks on arrival and as they age they have often a greater increased need for social support than long-term residents of an area. Those areas of the country with the highest proportion of older people include coastal areas, particularly the south coast and North Wales and attractive rural inland areas such as the Cotswolds, the Lake District, the Yorkshire Dales and mid-Wales and the Welsh Borders. Other areas, however, which formerly had a low proportion of elderly people such as the post-war suburbs of cities and towns are also showing an ageing profile (Law and Warnes, 1985). Migration of kin also effects those of us in later life who decide to stay put in an area with which we are familiar. With increasing geographical mobility in the general population close family may have often moved away from their area of origin in search of employment or a preferred lifestyle.

As an increasing proportion of people reaching retirement age are owner occupiers, retirement migration is likely to increase as older people realise their housing assets and retire to an area of the country where housing costs are lower and the area is more attractive. International migration is also showing an increase especially within the European Community. This trend may be moderated, however, by the problems associated with obtaining care and support in later life in places such as the south of Spain or the Greek islands.

Housing

In Britain some 95% of people of pensionable age live in private households, although in later life we are all likely to experience life in an institution of some kind. Of older people living in private households about 5% will live in some form of sheltered accommodation with a warden (Butler et al., 1983). Thus, about nine in ten elderly people live in general housing.

Historically elderly people have been less likely than younger people to own or be purchasing their own accommodation. Nevertheless, in line with general trends, the proportion of elderly people who are owner-occupiers has increased from about four-fifths in 1980 to over one half in 1988 (OPCS, 1982; 1990). There is a steady decline in owner occupation with increasing age. This is partly because some elderly people are realising their assets in order to pay for residential care or joining other households, but mainly because elderly people were less able or less inclined to buy their own property when they were younger.

Elderly people are more likely than younger people to live in older housing, which is likely to be in poorer condition, lacking in amenities and with sub-standard heating (OPCS, 1982). The 1986 English House Condition Survey (Department of Health, 1988) found that about 5% of the housing in England was unfit for habitation. Although accounting for only 10% of households, those where the head of household was 75 years of age or over occupied about one third of dwellings lacking basic amenities and some 16% of those unfit for habitation. The survey also found that elderly people living alone (19%) were more likely to occupy housing in poor condition than elderly couples (14%).

SPECIALIST HOUSING

Inadequate housing conditions can be particularly problematic for elderly people who are impaired, handicapped or disabled. A lack of adequate housing has been blamed for the unnecessary admission of older people into residential care (Townsend, 1986). The development of specialist housing for elderly people has been seen as the most appropriate solution although Butler et al (1983) concluded that sheltered housing created an elite whose housing needs were not different from those of the elderly population as a whole. One response to this study was the development of the policy of 'staying put'.

STAYING PUT

The policy of 'staying put' aims at helping elderly people remain in their own homes by providing a more flexible approach to addressing the housing needs of elderly people. It has come about through the activities of voluntary organisations, housing associations, building societies and local authorities, rather than central government. Tinker (1984) studied a number of schemes provided by local authorities and concluded that elderly people were satisfied with the schemes and the cost of the schemes. Income and housing costs were lower than for residential homes or sheltered housing. If the costs of informal care were added, however, both for sheltered housing and 'staying put' schemes, overall costs might rise above the costs of residential care.

Table 3.5: Household structure of elderly people

	1945[1]*	1962[1]	1976[1]	1980[1]	1989[2]
	%	%	%	%	%
Living alone	10	22	30	34	36
Living with spouse only	30	33	44	45	46
Living with others	60	44	27	22	18

* These data are not nationally representative

Sources:

1. *Dale, A., Evandrou, M. and Arber, S. (1987) 'The household structure of the elderly population in Britain',* Ageing and Society, *7, pp.37-56. Table 1.*
2. *Department of Health (1992)* The Health of Elderly People. An Epidemiological Overview. *London: HMSO. Table 4.*

Household structure

Demographic, economic and social factors have all combined to change the pattern of living arrangements of people in later life. Table 3.5 illustrates the dramatic nature of these changes, highlighting the decline in the proportion of the elderly population living with others. Among factors which have influenced this decline are the reduction in the average number of children and their earlier and more frequent marriage for the current cohort of elderly people; greater geographical mobility; the increase in employment opportunities for women over the last 20 years; and the improvement in the availability of housing for younger people since the war. The opportunity to express a general preference to live alone has been enabled by increasing personal resources. General Household Survey data show that the majority of elderly people live with a spouse, or after widowhood alone (Dale et al., 1987; Department of Health, 1992). Greater longevity among women than men means that they are more likely to be widowed and therefore live alone.

It is difficult to obtain a clear picture of the household structure of elderly people from ethnic minorities because of the paucity of data about elderly people from different ethnic communities. Local studies suggest that the household structure of elderly people in ethnic groups from outside Asia are similar to the general population. Older people from Asian communities are more likely to live with others (Bhalla and Blakemore, 1981).

In the future it is estimated by the Department of Environment that the number and proportion of single-person-pensioner

Figure 3.3 Long term care places in UK, 1970-1991

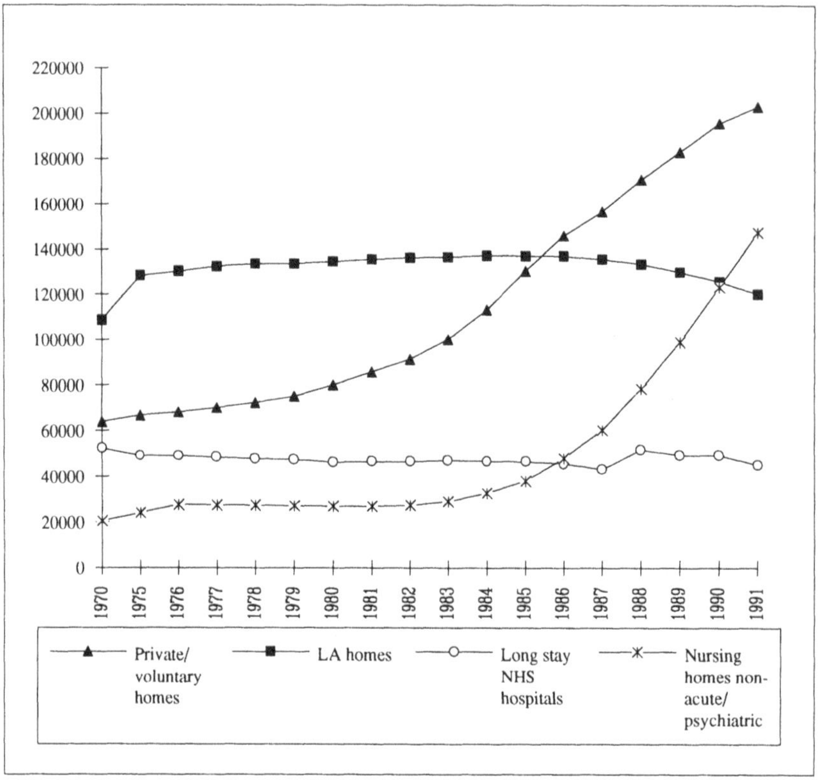

Source: Laing, W. & Buisson. (1992) *Laing and Buisson Review of Private Health Care.* London: Laing & Buisson. Table 4.2.

households will increase into the twenty-first century. The implications for housing and care policies of the increased number of single-pensioner households are substantial since single elderly people are likely to be older and more frail than the current cohort.

Institutional living

Throughout history a small proportion of elderly people have lived in an institution of some kind (Thomson, 1983). Remarkably since the establishment of the welfare state the proportion has remained constant with between 4 and 5% living permanently or temporarily in an institution (OPCS and Registrar General Scotland, 1983). As mental and physical frailty increased, so an elderly person is increasingly likely to experience institutional living. At the 1981 Census, 9.6% of people aged 75 years or over and 21.6% of people aged 85 years or over were resident in an institution on Census night.

During the 1980s there was a change in the types of institutional facilities available. As Figure 3.3 shows there was an increase in the provision of private residential and nursing-home places. The increase in demand for places was encouraged by the availability of income support throughout the 1980s (Secretaries of State for Health et al., 1989). The introduction of controls on funding for residential care in 1993 will probably reduce the increase in provision by the private sector. An alternative to residential care currently being explored by some housing associations is the development of very sheltered housing with extra-care services being provided to tenants rather than necessitating the transfer of a frail person to institutional care (Fletcher, 1991).

In the longer term we might expect that the control of the supply of residential and nursing home care by limiting the amount of money available to spend on institutional care will lead to only extremely frail people being cared for in institutions (Bond, 1992). It is very difficult to predict, however, whether this scenario will evolve. At present for every person exhibiting extreme frailty living in an institution there are at least three living in private households including sheltered housing facilities (Townsend and Wedderburn, 1965; Bond and Carstairs, 1982). Into the 21st century we can expect to continue to find a substantial number of extremely frail elderly people living outside institutional care.

Understanding living arrangements in later life

Old age has for many years been seen as a social problem (MacIntyre, 1977) and as we have observed this perspective has helped perpetuate ageism. As a result, in any discussion of living arrangements in later life there has usually been more emphasis on the current needs of frail elderly people than on the current and future needs of elderly people in general.

In understanding why an individual person has any one particular living arrangement it is important to understand the powerful role that their structural position in society at earlier stages in the life cycle plays. Owner-occupiers tend to remain owner-occupiers, council tenants tend to remain council tenants and private tenants tend to remain private tenants. People's lives in later life are strongly influenced by their access to resources and social goods throughout their lives. Housing tenure remains one of the most sensitive indicators of an individual's access to resources, although many elderly owner-occupiers lack the resources to keep their property in good repair. As owner-occupiers become older and more frail they have a disposable asset for the securing of a smaller or more appropriate dwelling than council or private tenants. In the event of requiring institutional care owner-occupiers could also use these resources to fund institutional care of their choice. Most elderly people, however, are not likely to require long-term care and will remain in their own homes for much of their later life.

SOCIAL NETWORKS

One of the myths about later life which remains prevalent today is the idea that the family will continue to play a dominant role in later life. Well-documented community studies of family life during the 1950s (Townsend, 1957; Young and Willmott, 1957) describe the close reciprocal relationships of families and concluded that elderly people were well integrated in family life. What was true in post-war Britain is increasingly incorrect as we enter the last decade of the century some forty years later. Of course, this vision of closely integrated families and thriving communities is central to government policy and the way so many centre-right politicians think. The Census data on household structure reported above and numerous recent studies of elderly people suggest otherwise. For example, in a national survey of later life in the 1970s Abrams (1978) uncovered a high level of loneliness and isolation among elderly people. Of course, even in close-knit communities like those in East London elderly people were lonely and hence the important distinction to be made between the concepts of loneliness and isolation (Townsend, 1957). Yet isolation increased as a result of a number of concurrent social changes, particularly changes in family size and family structure.

Changes in the family

Post-war housing developments helped to herald the destruction of traditional communities (Willmott and Young, 1960) but increased labour-force activity by women and greater geographical mobility as traditional heavy industries declined were also contributory factors to the increased isolation of people in later life. Increased isolation, however, has mainly been influenced by the structure of families. There are now far fewer children per elderly person as we move toward the close of the century than there were some 30-40 years ago. This reflects changes in family size which occurred much earlier in this century when family size decreased quite sharply.

In Victorian and Edwardian families it was not unusual for there to be six, seven or eight children. Many of the elderly people living in East London in the 1950s would have borne their children at the turn of the century. At this time children were more likely to survive than in previous generations because of the improvements in public hygiene, medical treatments and living conditions at the end of the nineteenth century. Thus although a large number of sons were lost during the 1914-18 war this had the consequence that there were later more single women available to care for their elderly relatives. In some respects, therefore, elderly people living in the 1950s were advantaged in ways not seen before and not repeated for later cohorts (Coleman et al., 1993). The solidarity of working-class communities during the 1950s was a positive product of urbanisation. In earlier periods of history there was probably less contact between families because travel was not so easy between rural communities.

The situation some forty years later is a very different one. After the 1914-18 war family size declined rapidly. As a consequence, about one quarter of surviving elderly people aged 75 years or over have no surviving children and about one-fifth no surviving siblings (Bond and Carstairs, 1982; Victor, 1987).

In addition to a decline in the size of families, the impact of divorce and remarriage, geographical mobility and changes in employment patterns has forced other changes in the structure of the family, particularly the provision of family support, although the extent of informal caregiving and support by family members is evidence to the continuing strength of the family (Parker, 1990). Yet changes in the family have undoubtedly resulted in the weakening of connections between the generations, where complex patterns of family relationships have often taken the place of simple ties. This is not to say that individual bonds of affection and responsibility between parents and their children have necessarily diminished. Other forms of intimate relationships have emerged for many elderly people, suggesting that contact with other than family members are relatively more important nowadays (Jerrome, 1993).

WORK AND RETIREMENT IN LATER LIFE

Perhaps one of the most important influences on an individual's later life, after the family, is their experience of work and retirement. Of course, when thinking about the work experiences of the current cohort of elderly people we must understand the significant gender differences. Men of this age group have usually been in paid employment whereas women may have only been on the margins of paid employment. Phillipson (1993), reporting economic activity rates, shows a substantial increase between 1971-91. Women, however, are more likely to work part time and to work in less skilled occupations (Dex, 1985). The traditional role of women was one of unpaid work and one which usually revolved around domestic labour (Graham, 1991).

Perspectives on retirement differ. Traditionally it was seen as a status passage which particularly affected men, since women were not perceived as major participants in the labour market. Retirement research from the last two decades suggests that this traditional view no longer holds. The important focus of recent research has been on the relationship between retirement and other phases in the life course, which has highlighted variations in experience of retirement, reflecting lifelong inequalities and differences produced by class, gender, ethnicity and health. Phillipson (1987) has concluded that the transition to retirement is not a change from an old to a completely new way of life but the final resolution of the advantages and disadvantages attached to a given gender and class position. For some people retirement enables them to consolidate their advantaged social position, while for others, who are disadvantaged, it increases an individual's sense of powerlessness in an intensely stratified society. From this perspective an individual's position in the world of work has profound influences on their experiences of later life.

STANDARDS OF LIVING IN LATER LIFE

In later life then, our standard of living will be influenced most markedly by our work experience although the quality of our social networks and state of health will also have some influence.

In 1978 the Royal Commission on the Distribution of Income and Wealth reported that one in three elderly families had incomes on or below the 'poverty line' in 1975 and that nearly three in every four lived on the margins of poverty (Walker, 1993). With the rise in owner-occupancy, increases in state pensions and the more general introduction of occupational

Table 3.6: Gross household income, 1989

Profile of households in gross weekly income groups

		Less than £80	Over £80 less than £175	Over £175
Single person households:				
Retired households mainly dependent on state pensions	%	70	29	1
Other retired households	%	4	57	39
Two person households:				
Retired households mainly dependent on state pensions	%	3	90	7
Other retired households	%	-	23	77

Source*: Central Statistical Office (1992)* Family Spending. A Report on the 1991 Family Expenditure Survey. *London: HMSO. Table 22.*

pension schemes, there is a general belief that current cohorts of elderly people are better off. For a minority there is evidence that this is indeed the case but for the majority later life is a time of lowering standards of living.

Routinely published statistics from the Family Expenditure Survey (FES) provide information about the incomes of elderly-person households. Table 3.6 shows estimates of gross income of different types of households from the 1991 FES compiled by the Central Statistical Office (CSO, 1992). Elderly-person households (referred to as pensioner households) have much lower incomes than non-pensioner households. For example, in 1989 the mean income of all pensioner households was £99.88 per week, but the median income was less than £75; 70% of pensioner households having less than the average. At the top end of the income distribution only 10% of pensioner households had an income in excess of £150 per week (CSO, 1990).

Sources of income

In 1989 42% of the income of elderly people came, on average from state benefits. Although a minority of elderly people receive a higher income with contributions from an occupational pension, investment income and savings income, and other sources, the majority are still mainly dependent on the State Retirement Pension and other benefits. Figure 3.4 (see p.62) illustrates the

Figure 3.4 Pensioners' incomes by quintile showing sources of income in 1987

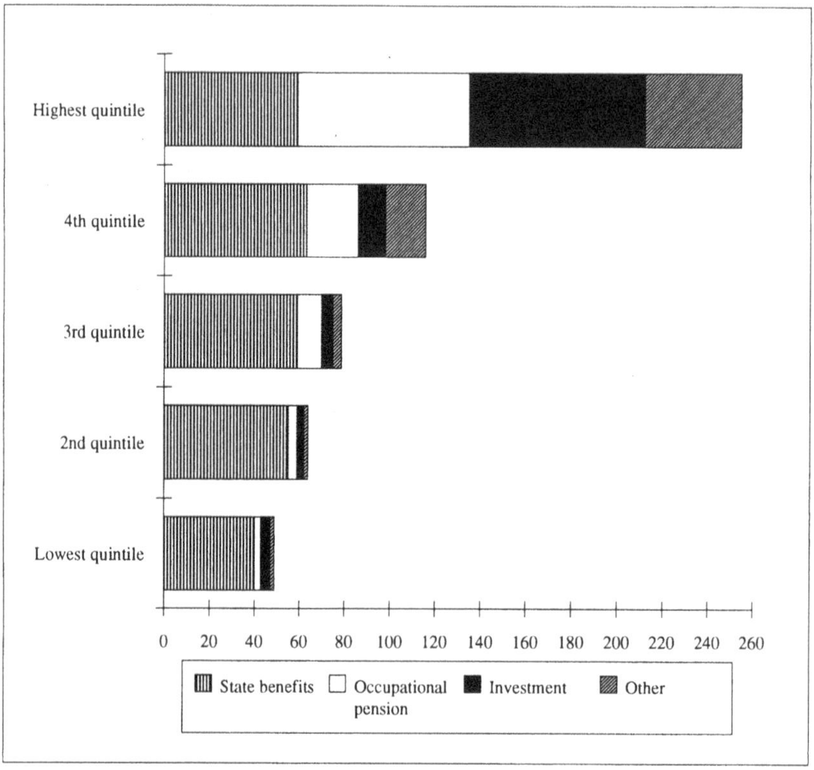

Source: House of Commons (1990). *Parliamentary Debates (Hansard). Sixth Series, Volume 177.* London: HMSO. Table 3.

contribution of different sources of incomes of elderly people within quintiles of gross weekly income. It is only in the highest quintile (the top 20% of incomes) that other sources of income to state benefits account for more than half.

DEPRIVATION AND POVERTY

The high incidence of poverty and low incomes among elderly people is reflected in other measures of deprivation. Townsend (1979) shows, for example, that elderly people have less consumer durables of their own than younger people, are less likely to eat fresh meat and are less likely to take a summer holiday. We have already seen that elderly people are less likely to be owner-occupiers and when they are so they live in dwellings which lack one or more basic amenities.

AGEING WELL IN LATER LIFE

In considering the social context of later life this chapter has identified two key ideas. First, that elderly people are relatively disadvantaged in modern Europe because of institutionalised ageism. But, second, the enormous diversity of experience of elderly people has been noted. This experience is very much determined by experiences of earlier stages in the life course. Thus inequalities in later life are primarily a function of access to resources when younger. Occupational status in earlier life determines income levels and, thereafter, the ability to save and invest in property and other possessions. Occupational class, gender, ethnic origin and health status all influence the individual's experience of later life. In addition, cohort experiences such as major wars, economic recession and major social change will all have some affect on an individual's own attitude toward later life.

The theoretical perspective which links these ideas together is that of political economy using the concept of structured dependency (Townsend, 1981; 1986; Walker, 1982; Walker and Phillipson, 1986). This can be most clearly seen through Phillipson's analysis of retirement (Phillipson, 1982, 1993). Prior to retirement skilled and semi-skilled employees experience reduced economic status (Townsend, 1979). Increasingly early retirement schemes are pushing older workers into less skilled employment and into unemployment. After retirement the inequalities resulting from low pay, unemployment, disability, and for women and ethnic minorities, sex and race discrimination, are carried forward into later life. The decline in the real value of savings and pensions means that the very old are the worse off. Retirement also restricts access to social resources in the form of a reduction in social relationships once the retiree is away from the world of work.

What relevance does this have to the world of social care? Many elderly people who use social care services will be disadvantaged by their lack of financial resources and therefore their relative powerlessness. Structural dependency also highlights the way that statutory services restrict the freedom of the individual to determine his or her own course of action, because the receiver is usually in a subordinate position to the provider. This is perhaps most clearly illustrated by reference to institutional care.

The social context of later life and institutional care

Many institutions in the United Kingdom, existing for the care of elderly people, exhibit a number of the characteristics of what Goffman (1961) termed the total institution. Goffman's description of the total institution as an abstract concept has dominated much of our thinking in the last thirty years to such an extent that we are all likely to be guilty of accepting the inevitableness of the characteristics described. The essential feature of the total institution as described by Goffman is that, unlike life outside, there is no separation between the three central spheres of modern life: work, leisure and family. All aspects of life are conducted within the boundaries of the institution and under the control of a single authority. Each phase of daily activities is shared with a large number of other people, all of whom are treated alike and are required to do the same things together. These activities normally follow a strict routine imposed from above by a system of explicit formal rulings and a body of officials. The routine of daily activities comprises a single rational plan which has been designed to fulfil the official aims of the institution.

The extreme nature of Goffman's description, which he also applied to prisons and monasteries as well as psychiatric hospitals, might be questioned by many workers providing care to elderly people in residential settings on the grounds that many of these characteristics are not exhibited in their institution. Yet the consistency of findings from studies of residential and hospital care for elderly people and chronically sick and disabled people support the value of Goffman's analysis which shows how institutionalised ageism and the disadvantaged position of elderly people in society can be reinforced in an institutional setting during later life.

Townsend's (1962) study of residential care in England and Wales remains, after over thirty years the best description of the ubiquity of the total institution. His case studies of residents in old work houses, which provided the mainstay of local authority residential services for elderly and disabled people, vividly describe the isolation of residents from the outside world, the lack of individual privacy and independence, the routinisation of activities, and the separation of residents from staff.

Although much of the physical conditions described by Townsend no longer exist with the development of purpose built homes for elderly people the legacy of the workhouse often continues within the organisational culture of residential settings. Miller and Gwynne (1972), Booth (1985) and Willcocks et al. (1987) in their studies of residential homes and Baker (1978), Evers (1981), Clark and Bowling (1989) and Bond and Bond (1990) in their studies of hospital wards for elderly people have identified the continuing existence of many of the characteristics of the total institution described by Goffman. As Booth concludes differences between residential homes should 'be seen as a veneer that decorates the massive uniformity of institutional life.... Underneath lies the same crushing panoply of controls over the lives and doings of residents. Changing the wrapper does not alter the contents.' (Booth, 1985, p.206).

Changing the institutional culture

How do we change the contents of residential care and overcome the effects of institutionalised ageism? We can begin by learning from this analysis. First we should remember that every elderly person has a unique biography and we should not typify individuals according to ageist stereotypes. Understanding their personal history and responding positively to it will encourage personal fulfilment for some of our most vulnerable citizens. Second, we should understand that elderly people are disadvantaged by their structural position in society. This does not sanction us to infantilise elderly people nor does it give us the authority to ignore their perspective on life. As individuals we will be equally vulnerable unless we all work together to change the culture and challenge institutionalised ageism.

One way we can all do this is to challenge our own attitudes. In their study of people with physical disabilities Dartington et al. (1981) identified a number of attitudinal constructs held by providers of care. Do you recognise any of these in yourself?

'The less than whole person' construct reflects the view that because people are physically or mentally frail and probably socially isolated they are assumed to have lost the right to be autonomous human beings. The opportunity for having choices is further dissipated by group living and the institution of routines. This construct is one which has been observed to be held by staff in many studies of institutional care for elderly people.

'The really normal' construct, which represents the liberal challenge to the total institution, places greater emphasis on the individual's rights to dignity, choice, privacy and the maintenance of independence even where residents require substantial support from others. As a result the autonomy needs are met and the difference between normal, able-bodied people and disabled people are denied, so that the need for physical and emotional support may be unmet.

Recognition of both autonomy and physical and emotional needs are recognised in the third attitudinal construct 'Enlightened Guardianship'. While this attitude summarises the position of staff towards residents it requires that the latter are expected to adjust to their impairments and dependency in return for enlightened treatment. This attitudinal construct would reject the infantilism of 'Less Than Whole Person' so that staff remove the autonomy and reinforce the dependency of residents.

The fourth attitudinal construct is 'Disabled Power' which heightens the political consciousness of the disabled group by asserting their differences from others. It is contrasted with 'Really Normal' which asserts sameness with the majority and 'Enlightened Guardianship' which emphasises adjustment to societal norms. 'Disabled Power' unlike the other three constructs emanated from disabled people themselves rather than from care staff. It emphasises rights rather than privileges and reflects able-bodied values in respect of disabled people while asserting that to be different is positive. 'Disabled Power' is thus in opposition to the other three constructs and so cannot mediate relationships between disabled people and others, except in confrontation.

Frail elderly people who assert themselves are unlikely to have accepted residential care in the first place and will organise their support and manage at home. Older people who are so frail that they or their family are unable to cope at home are unlikely to be able to function in residential care through 'Disabled Power'. They would refuse to adjust to the routines of the institution and others' definitions of what is realistic and in so doing be branded 'Less Than Whole Person'. Dartington et al. (1981) advocate transactions between disabled people and others which accepts their dependency needs without giving up their personal autonomy in their daily lives. In this analysis, however, to accept dependency needs means giving up autonomy since even in 'Enlightened Guardianship' it is staff who believe themselves to be enlightened, to know best and to define appropriate adjustment to disability.

In recognising a particular attitude construct in oneself there is the natural tendency to argue that one is constrained by the institutional environment. To some extent this will be true. In a truly total institution the lives of staff are as controlled as much as are the lives of residents. Yet in enlightened organisations where some senior staff may be attempting to change the culture a number of attitudinal constructs may be held by different members of staff, who may unaware of the attitudes they hold.

Take infantilism for example. Many staff do not recognise that they are infantilising residents. Recently I had the privilege, as part of a research study, to interview an elderly lady of 87 years in hospital five days after she had suffered a severe stroke. She appeared particularly depressed, a not unusual reaction for a relatively active person to experience on becoming disabled. As a visiting research worker I had time to spend talking to this lady and because I was interested in her, I was able to establish a good rapport. A few days later I was visiting the same ward and took the opportunity to spend a few minutes renewing our acquaintance. I was introduced by the young nurse as her 'boyfriend'. The nurse was well meaning who under the pressures of a very busy ward was attempting to cheer up the patient. She did not think that it was abnormal to introduce two comparative strangers in this way. Yet it is the kind of remark one might usually make within one's family in relation to young teenagers.

By understanding one's own attitude we are all in a position to challenge the way we relate to clients as well as to other members of staff in order to move toward 'Enlightened Guardianship'. In understanding the social context of ageing we should all be better placed to recognise the way in which many of us reinforce institutionalised ageism in everyday life.

Perhaps the first step in making a change in the organisational culture is to challenge the way staff refer to and talk about clients. Like sexism and racism, ageism is difficult to overcome since we are often socialised into thinking and acting in ways which are offensive to older people, women and people from ethnic minorities. Yet the challenge is one that we should all except in order that some of our most vulnerable fellow citizens can live the last years of their lives in dignity and respect.

Four:

Housing and services for older people

Roger Clough

INTRODUCTION

This chapter starts with a discussion of the types of housing in which older people live, the reasons for their living in those particular places and the problems which emerge. The focus shifts for the remainder of the chapter to those older people who, on account of some difficulty in managing on their own, want or need a combination of appropriate housing and appropriate services.

The context of the discussion is crucia:

> Old people are, compared with the rest of the population, more likely to be disabled, poor, badly housed and widowed. Moreover, an elderly person who suffers one of these disadvantages is more likely to suffer one of the others. The disadvantages, singly, or more damagingly in combination, affect the ability of elderly people to live their lives as they wish (Sinclair et al., 1990, p.367).

To this should be added, as Williams (1990) points out, the fact that 'black and minority ethnic elders generally do experience "triple jeopardy", that is cumulative disadvantage in addition to the disadvantages faced by other older people':

> ...they suffer the effects of racism; they are disadvantaged in housing, health, employment and pensions; and services are not tailored to their general and specific needs (Williams, 1990, p.134).

Williams acknowledges the difficulty, because of the lack of comparability of data, in interpreting some statistics on racial differences; she points out also that there are substantial differences, as will emerge later, between different black and minority ethnic groups in terms of numbers of home owners and numbers of older people living alone.

However, in addition, for people who were not born in the UK, we have little information of what it is like to grow old and face dying in a land which is not your birthplace. We know about the significance of reviewing the present in the context of the past– but not how this is managed by people who were immigrants.

Two thirds of older people over 75 years of age are women. They are more likely than men to live alone. They have to manage their attitudes to past stereotyping and live with present stereotyping, in which they are expected to assume certain roles. In addition, they may feel frightened of attack. We have to remember that the overwhelming majority of people providing services are also women.

THE PLACE WHERE PEOPLE LIVE

There have been three broad categories of housing in which older people live: ordinary housing; special housing; residential institutions:

- *ordinary housing*: by the term 'ordinary housing' I am referring to the types of housing which are generally available to or used by the whole of the population, whatever their age. Such housing may be in the form of bungalow, house or flat.
- *special housing*: frequently known as sheltered housing, the characteristic of this type of housing is that it has been built with a purpose of providing appropriate facilities, including access to alarm systems and support.
- *residential institutions*: this category includes residential homes, nursing homes and hospitals. I use the word 'institution' in a neutral sense to describe a building in which a number of people live who are brought together because of a common characteristic, in this context that of a need or want for services to help them manage their daily lives. I am not implying that residential homes necessarily run in an institutional way, in the pejorative sense of the word.

In any one of these categories there are four key dimensions:

- *ownership*: people may be owners (in part or outright) or tenants (of public, private or voluntary providers);

- *quality*: basic amenities, state of repair, ease of maintenance, security;
- *location*: rural or urban; access to shops or transport; safety of environment;
- *nature of household*: living alone or with others (with partner, children, other family, others not related).

Trends

There has been a significant increase in the number of owner occupiers, in the variety of types of special housing and, within the institutional sector, an expansion of private residential and nursing homes accompanied by a decrease in local authority homes and in long stay hospital beds.

Most passion has been spent on who should be the providers of residential institutions. The more significant longer term development is the merging of former boundaries between the three types of housing listed above. Thus, there is an increasing number of retirement flatlets, some built as what has been termed 'very sheltered housing' with facilities which are designed to allow someone to stay until he or she would have to go into hospital, that is the stage at which a residential home would have to be left. These houses may be under private, voluntary (often housing association) or local authority ownership. What is significant about these is the amount of space people have compared to a traditional residential home: typically, such a small house or flatlet has a kitchen and a sitting room (or a kitchen diner), one or two bedrooms and a bathroom; as important, the house has its own front door. The feel is that of people living in their own house and of others coming in to provide services.

Discussions of the respective costs of residential home and services provided to people in their own homes too often have ignored the housing cost that is contained within the residential home fee. Such debate has also largely ignored the conflict created by setting up home ownership as a mark of successful life style and then requiring older people to spend this asset on the purchase of a place in a residential home. The housing capital is transferred from individual older people to the owners of a private home or to the local authority. Not surprisingly, there is resentment abut such payment.

In considering trends we have to be aware also of improvements in housing standards. In ordinary housing the most significant have been:

- the increase in the number of bathrooms and indoor WCs;
- central heating and insulation;
- the ratio of rooms per household member.

Within residential institutions the most significant development since the 1950s has been that the huge, workhouse type buildings have been almost eliminated and, in the present smaller homes, there is an increase in the number of single as opposed to multi occupancy rooms, with some of these including en suite WCs and washing facilities.

I have no doubt that we should be planning to abolish all traditional residential institutions except hospitals by the year 2020 so that the minimum standard for an older person in any setting is a flatlet. This has immense advantages: the place is not necessarily the property of the people providing services and each resident has an amount of space more in keeping with what she or he has been used to. I am not arguing that flatlets should not be placed together, which might be seen as a residential community rather than a residential institution. I want older people who require services to be assured of a better standard of housing than residential institutions supply.

HOUSING SEPARATED FROM SERVICES

Linked to this crossing of boundaries of housing types is a shift in analysis of functions which envisages a separation of housing from service provision.

In considering the range of services which could be offered to someone it is helpful to separate a housing component from a care component. The tendency has been to offer people packages of care which have arisen from structures within or between organisations. One of the most significant aspects of the Wagner Report is the backing it gives to a much clearer analysis of functions. Those who want care support will have a need for first housing and secondly for services. (Clough and Parsloe, 1989, p.16)

The National Health Service and Community Care Act 1989, drawing heavily on the Griffiths report, creates a structure in which local authorities are given the authority to assess the care needs of individual people who want state financial support. This is to be followed by an attempt to match the assessment with what is available, with the individual getting the maximum feasible amount of control and choice. Someone, usually known in the literature as the care manager, has the responsibility for translating plan into reality.

The intention is that there should be a break with a former pattern of state services in which the choice for many people was between minimal services at home and maximal services in a residential home. The new system should allow people to have individualised packages of care in the place that suits them best. Thus someone who wants help with getting to the lavatory twice during the day and with getting into bed at night time *and* wants to stay in her or his own home, should be able to get it. The package of care is designed to take account of the person's capacity and of the various caring networks. However, there are inevitable limitations: the costs of individualised care at home may overtake those of a residential home; the staff or services that are wanted may not be able to be found; the total costs of services wanted by people may exceed the amount allocated.

As Griffiths (1988) suggested the proposals:

> ...will increase the ability of managers in all community care services to ensure that:
> • the right services are provided in good time, to the people who need them most;
> • the people receiving help will have a greater say in what is done to help them, and a wider choice;
> • people are helped to stay in their own homes for as long as possible, or in as near a domestic environment as possible, so that residential, nursing home and hospital care is reserved for those whose needs cannot be met in any other way(p.28).

Wagner (1988) sets out various principles:

> People who move into residential establishments should do so by positive choice. A distinction should be made between need for accommodation and need for services. No one should be required to change their permanent accommodation in order to receive services which could be made available to them in their own homes (p.114).

The new systems envisage also that local authorities will not necessarily provide as much care as formerly. Their task is to assess people for care and then to purchase the appropriate care, which may be provided by the local authority sector itself or by the independent sector, made up of voluntary organisations and privately managed homes and agencies. And so we move into the brave new world of 'purchaser' and 'provider'.

THE PLACES WHERE PEOPLE LIVE AND THEIR CIRCUMSTANCES

People are more likely to need state support for services in old age if their present housing is poor, if they become incapacitated, if they have little money and if they live alone, particularly if they live some distance from their children.

The graph that has shown a steady rise in the total numbers of very old people is flattening. Projections suggest that between 1971 and 2001 the number of people aged over 65 years who live alone will increase by 29%, the number unable to get in or out of bed without help will rise from 122,000 to 185,000 (52%) and the number of people suffering from dementia will increase from 450,000 to 684,000 (again 52%). This is largely explained by the rise in numbers of people aged over 85 years, which was expected to more than double in the same period. (Sinclair, 1990, p.24 adapted from Henwood and Wicks, 1984)

A study of the household structures of people over 65 years shows that nearly a half live as part of a couple, about one third live on their own, 10% live as single elderly people with younger household members and a further 8% live as a couple with younger household members (Sinclair, 1990, p.26 from Evandrou et al., 1986). It should be noted that only about 10% of older people want to live with their children, though most want to live close to them.

Williams (1990, p.111) states: 'Nationally, the proportion of 'pensioner only' households among the West Indian and Asian population is very low (2.3% when compared with the 'white' population (29%) (Brown, 1984)'. She shows from different studies that only 4% to 5% of older people of Asian and Indian origin live alone, in contrast with the 33% for the total population of older people. It is frequently assumed that older people of Asian and Indian origin will have extended families which will share in their care. Some studies, such as those of Fenton in Bristol (1986), show that only about a quarter live in extended households.

The patterns of where people live is important because there has been increasing evidence that neighbours and friends are unlikely to provide intimate personal care (Power et al., 1983; Levin et al., 1989; Sinclair et al., 1988)). The latter is particularly useful in showing that older people themselves are willing to have particular sorts of help only from particular sorts of people. The pattern that emerges is that spouses do provide intimate care of their partners, with children doing so less often. Whether or not intimate, personal care is provided is dependent on the willingness of one person to provide the care and on another to receive it. Fathers are more likely to receive care from daughters than are mothers from sons, for both of these reasons. Neighbours and friends may provide emergency surveillance and occasional shopping but are unlikely to provide personal care, affection or even discussions of matters that worry older people. It would appear that there is no substitute for certain personal services being provided by a paid worker who is acceptable by virtue of the fact that she or he is a stranger.

MOVING HOME IN OLD AGE

There are two main patterns of housing move in old age: the first is that of people moving immediately after retirement; the second is people who stay in their existing home until they are unable to cope.

Karn (1977) discusses the first of these in studying people who retired to the seaside. She explodes the myth that such people are doomed to unhappiness: over three quarters were pleased with the move (pp.242-43). Most moved as couples, though after death of a spouse, many moved again. The people who moved to the seaside were likely to have less strong links with children and nearly all were owner occupiers. They moved for what they judged a better way of life: more peace and a healthier environment.

Older people want to move home for the obvious pull of a new place and for the equally obvious wish to avoid problems of looking after a house and garden which was may be larger than needed. Some hope to purchase cheaper property so that they may use some of their capital. The potential for mobility is hugely greater for owners than tenants and there is thus a big class bias in who is able to make these sorts of choices.

Moving to a new area where few if any people are known presents risks of isolation. The probability is that people who make these moves successfully are those who move with someone else and do so soon after retirement. It is also likely that the expectations and psychological state of people are significant: For example, in her study of Sussex towns to which people retire, Karn found that people's social contacts were largely with older couples: those who were on their own or who wanted contacts with younger people were more likely to be dissatisfied.

The greater the incapacity to care for self, the greater the likelihood that a person will be in a hospital rather than a nursing home, or a nursing home rather than a residential care home. Alongside this is the fact that more people with severe disabilities and minimal capacity to care for self live at home than live in these same institutions.

Bebbington and Tong (1986), drawing on figures from the early 1980s, show that of older people with the highest levels of incapacity, 9,000 live on their own, 78,000 live with others and only 24,000 in residential care. Even when allowances are made for the recent growth in the numbers of nursing homes and for attaching some credence to the claim that today residents are more incapacitated than previously, the information is stark. Three times as many older people with high levels of incapacity live outside residential homes as live within them.

LIFE SATISFACTION AND DECISION-MAKING IN OLD AGE

The reasons for making particular decisions and their likelihood of being successful are numerous and may be interconnected. Gubrium (1973) suggests that the most important factor is a match between resources and expectations:

- *resources:* personal resources in terms of money and health; external resources such as the quality and the ease of management of the environment (for example the type of house or the nearness of shops and services, security, transport); other important external resources are people, perhaps friends, neighbours or relatives and services such as chiropody, home care, nursing and provision of meals.
- *expectations - 'personal, class or cultural':* a part of the reason why people make decisions is related to the norms as well as the hopes and dreams of people with whom they have grown up and with whom they live.

Gubrium considers that satisfaction in old age is related to the extent to which there is a match between the resources people have and the expectations that are held by themselves and important others. Thus, two people with similar resources in terms of housing and health will vary in the extent to which they feel satisfied in their lives with their own and others' expectations of how they ought to be living.

It is apparent also that circumstances may change rapidly as people get older, and that the capacity of any of us to cope may not be as great as we would wish. Tobin and Lieberman's (1976) study suggested that it was cumulative loss in a short space of time rather than particular personality types which made people less likely to live in a non domestic setting. Thus, an older person who is coping well may be faced with successive problems in personal health, the death of a partner and the moving away of a daughter or son. The authors' contention is that such losses render us more vulnerable than we may like to imagine.

Yet I think also that there is a danger in asserting the importance of things that happen to us and of minimising factors related to personality. The reality is that there is an interplay between personality and life events and that each of us has to decide on our own understanding of that interplay. This is an aspect of the nature or nurture debate as to why we are as we are. But it is essential also that our perspective is challenged by that of others and that we realise that others act on different beliefs than ours. We must avoid stereotypes, our own and others', of ageing as well as other categorisations.

I want to add a postscript to this discussion. Erikson (1950) writes of life stages at which people have to reach resolutions appropriate to that stage of development. In old age he writes of 'ego integrity versus despair'. Life events at different times in our lives may threaten our stability, our pictures of ourselves and our capacity to cope. What is significant in old age is both that such life events are more common and that we know that with most of our life lived, the fact of death is not far off. We find ourselves caught back in struggles that are related to previous life stages as well as those of our present.

I have suggested that choices are influenced by experiences, by expectations, by resources and by personal, internal state. This helps us to understand that some people stay happily in their current locality in old age, and others make the move, equally happily, to a new life in their dream house. Others are unhappy in either of these settings.

Susan Hill (1989) writes in her novel, *A Change for the Better*, of the struggles of a number of people to be themselves, a struggle which moves between what seems a proper and an improper self-centredness. One character, Mrs Carpenter, lives in a hotel with her husband after his retirement. He dies. Mrs Carpenter's response shocks people around her:

> 'I will not give way to old age and death', she said in a firm voice, 'I will not go into a decline and live off the kindness of others because I am now a widow. No, I have quite decided to take myself in hand at once' (p.188).

Another thinks that 'it is unseemly for her to come into this shop so full of excitement, looking so well and happy, when her husband is not three weeks dead'. But that person does not know of Mrs Carpenter's resolution about a new and active life, did not know of the long nights when she lay awake in her room ... and thought of how her husband had died. He was alone, she said to herself, a hundred times a day, he was alone, there was nobody to help. He was alone. At night Mrs Flora Carpenter wept, but she said nothing about any of it aloud, nothing to anyone (p.190).

My point is that we do not know how we will cope with events in our lives, nor can we know of the struggles of others. We know so much and yet so little about ourselves; however close to another, we know so little as well as so much.

One factor that does seem significant is that of degree of control: people are more likely to be contented with a decision which affects them when they have had an influence on that decision.

LIMITATIONS OF RESEARCH DATA

The discussion has focused on people planning in old age for their housing and for services. In doing so they take account of their own and others' views of what they should be doing. Some people, most likely those with more resources, plan for old age, though comparatively few plan for their potential incapacity. One of the aspects of ageing that has to be managed is that of an increased unpredictability. We know that people will become less able to do things for themselves and that people will die; we do not know the ways in which we will become incapacitated or whether we will die before spouse or close friends. There are limitations to planning.

A proviso has to be written in. The material in the earlier section on life satisfaction is developed from studies of white populations, largely in the USA. There is little written about the way in which black people and those from other minority ethnic groups make sense of their life history or of what is successful ageing. This has particular significance for people who in their generation were immigrants: how do they reconcile themselves to the prospect of dying and being buried in a country which is not the one in which they were born and grew up?

There are factors which are common to everybody faced with change; but there are issues, some of which were touched on earlier, which are specific to moving house in old age. Moving house is known to be one of the most significant situations of stress and has particular connotations in old age both because of the probability that this may be the last house in which people live and because it is less easy to manage many of the problems of moving: sorting out the old and the new place is harder when people are frail, have little money and less ability to control what has to be done.

In effect, little is known about the way in which certain attributes influence the common problems: getting to know people in a new place; living alone; moving into a residential home where you are dependent on others for service; living in a place which is not yours; living with others whom you have not chosen and with whom you do not necessarily have anything in common. This lack of knowledge is compounded by the need to know how these events are different for different people: women and men, people from different races and cultures, people with disabilities.

BEHAVIOUR IN INSTITUTIONS

I shall focus now on an understanding of behaviour in settings where people live some parts of their lives alongside others, typically a day or residential centre. Except for residential schools, few people dream about living in an institution and there are not even many who plan for it because they consider that it is their best alternative in the circumstances. Most want to avoid residential life. Sinclair (1988b) sums up the main criticisms of residential care:

> ...they are not places in which residents can be expected to live normal or reasonable lives...Few people want to go into residential care ...Traditional forms of residential care have proved ineffective...Residential care is usually more costly than possibly superior community provision catering for a similar clientele (p.46).

There is substantial evidence of the indignities of institutional life. As I have discussed elsewhere, these indignities are put alongside a myth of the golden years of old age to produce an irrefutable argument that life must be better outside residential homes (Clough, 1981, pp.8–15). The reality is that many older people living in their own homes are poor, lonely and in bad housing. The contrast is not between a miserable life in a residential home and an easy independence in one's own home.

There is a tendency in those who discuss residential care to place themselves or others into camps: in the one corner the 'residentialists', telling us of the potential of residential life; in the other, the 'home sweet homeists' who are certain that nobody should ever move into a residential home. Residential life at policy or practice level will never be satisfactory until the special characteristics of that life are understood. That real picture, not surprisingly, has greater complexity and subtlety.

I have already suggested that residential homes in their current form of large buildings with residents having at best individual bed sitting rooms will disappear over the next thirty years. The issue for the present is to improve practice so that the life style for residents is as good as can be achieved. One aspect of this is to understand processes.

The processes which are discussed here are those related to living in institutions: there are aspects of the same processes at work in relationships between service provider and individual.

People like Goffman whom I term the institutional theorists have had a major influence in analysing residential life. Their work, best studied in Jones and Fowles (1984), should be seen as *institutional tendencies* rather than absolutes. Thus when Goffman (1961) makes points about people being stripped (literally and psychologically) when they move into residential homes, the temptation for residential workers is to defend their place along the lines of 'He was writing about large establishments and our home is not like that'. It is right that not all residential establishments are like Goffman's stereotype. Nevertheless, I think it essential to acknowledge the tendency, even in small homes:

- for people to be stripped of (or to lose) their identity when they move in;
- for residents to feel powerless;
- for people's privacy to be invaded;
- for residents and carers to seem to be on opposite sides, as 'us' and 'them';
- for it to be easier to care for people in groups than separately;
- for people to be more vulnerable and less willing to criticise when they are dependent on others, (whether for care, money or somewhere to live) and when they have limited contact outside the residential home;

- for residents not to have chosen to live with the particular other people who live in the home;
- for there to be uncertainty about what people (both residents and staff) should expect of each other in terms of interaction and responsibilities;
- for the difficulties and unpleasantness of the job to be forgotten;
- for some workers to be attracted into the work because of the power that they may exert over others;
- for others to find the task beyond them and end up controlling residents in ways they would have found unacceptable when they started.

These points, not all taken from the institutional theorists, show that there are factors in both the nature of residential life and the nature of tending which create tendencies or pressures for people to behave in certain ways. There is no inevitability about this: good workers ensure that their systems and structures work against these pressures.

At the heart of these points are issues about the nature of the work, power and self.

THE PROVISION OF PERSONAL SERVICES

Parsloe (1989) distinguishes:

> ...caring for someone, in the sense of providing for their basic physical needs and caring about someone, by which we mean that the person feels love, affection, liking or concern ... for the other person, but does not necessarily do anything for them; and a combination of caring for and caring about (p.76).

She follows Parker (1981) in using the word 'tending' to describe the task of providing for someone's physical needs. Her analysis allows us to see one of the dilemmas of residential work. People live in homes because they need 'tending'. It is possible:

> ...to attend to someone gently and respectfully without loving or liking them for themselves, and it is possible for such attention to be acceptable to the person who receives it (Parsloe, 1989, p.79).

There are aspects of tending that are common whatever the setting. The more unhappy or insecure the person, the more she or he will look for affection from the worker. We know that in relationships the management of power and dependency is significant. We are used to the pack of cards which comprises our personal and work relationships, to dealing the cards and to being dealt them, and even to managing to play hands that we wished we had not got. When it comes to having help with personal tasks, it is not simply that the cards have been shuffled; they are different cards. Yet we will want the same things from them as we do in other aspects of our lives. In some way each of us has to get sufficient satisfaction in our interaction with others–and not all of us are as well able as Mrs Carpenter in the earlier extract to examine our position with reason and feeling and to act on what we find.

There is no single model of what the nature of the relationship should be between worker and individual. Sinclair and colleagues (1988) met older people who wanted their home care workers to know the way that they wanted the place looked after, and did not want to have to keep saying things to them. We all know how difficult it is to say things to others who are providing services in situations such as a hotel where there is little at stake. How much harder, whether for ourselves or those we love, when we are dependent on the worker both for the carrying out of the task and for the manner in which it is done.

Power is central to daily activities in all types of centres. Whose place is it? Who decides what people will do, what people will eat, the times of bathing and similar arrangements? Who is involved in drawing up care plans? How far can one group of people decide what is good for others and act on their conclusions? (Brown and Clough, 1989, p.5).

If we start from acknowledging the tensions, the difficult nature of the job and the complexities of staff motivation, we have a better hope of planning and producing good enough services in any setting. The task is not to make people happy: it is to tend others in ways which will not demean them and which allow for spontaneity and a measure of affection. To accomplish this, staff must understand the fragility of self image of many residents and must know the characteristics of good tending. As Parsloe (1989) stresses:

> ...what can be created is the knowledge of how to tend and the behaviour which usually accompanies affection: a willingness to spend time, to listen and to show an interest as well as to share something of oneself (p.81).

In *Old Age Homes* (Clough, 1981), I have tried to capture the confusions inherent in residential work with older people.

Staff working in old people's homes are at the centre of society's uncertainty about the purpose of such institutions. They are left to carry out a confused task in the way that they think best; in addition they are left to carry a mass of feelings from a multitude of people. They will be seen as saints and as sinners (p.139).

Staff want (and may be expected) to make residents happy– but many residents are too weary or bitter for happiness. 'Staff are faced with constant reminders of the harsher side of ageing' (p.140), and thus faced with thoughts of their futures. 'How will I or my family cope in similar circumstances?' they may well ask. The work itself is at times physically exhausting and, not to put too fine point on it, nasty: people who may be little able to help themselves have to be lifted and washed, the sorts of jobs parents have done with more or less love for children, staff do for adult strangers. Residential work encompasses the heaviest, perhaps least satisfying, aspects of housework, a task that inside and outside residential homes is predominantly undertaken by women. The task never seems finished: the tidy room will be made untidy, the person who is clean will become dirty.

There is no model for staff who work in such centres, in the way that there is for teaching or nursing. Of course people have widely different views on how to teach or the nature of the proper relationship between nurse and patient. But there is a picture which comes to people's minds of what these workers do. Managers and staff in day and residential centres are part caring relative (the good parent or child), part nurse, part domestic, part therapist, part friend.

If there is confusion about the nature of the task, there will be confusion for everybody. So clarification about what the worker should be doing is imperative for training and for practice.

GOOD PRACTICE

I shall focus now on good practice in settings where people live some parts of their lives alongside others, typically a day or residential centre. Good practice is influenced by values, by knowledge and by skills. Values, whether of agency, staff or residents often are not made explicit: when they are not, there is no bedrock to provide the solidity for the way people work, nor indeed to test the quality of that work. Knowledge enables staff to work better because they understand better. The skills referred to here are those of the staff, the techniques which they use to create a culture or life style and to carry out tasks.

The importance of agreement within the staff group about values comes from two contrasting sources. The first is that of literature on residential work with Wolins (1974) arguing that one of the characteristics of successful residential care is a shared value system. I have emphasised the dangers of fundamental, and often unacknowledged, staff disagreements about values and therefore the importance of specifying common values. (Clough, 1982, p.45) I think that conflicts about what should be included in a list of values would be few. The fundamental task is to capture what any of us would want for ourselves or others who need support to manage their lives: a respect for the individuality of each person, the right and opportunity for each person to make as many decisions as possible for him or herself, and so on.

Peters and Waterman (1982) and Peters and Austin (1985), in a study of the characteristics of the most successful American businesses, have put shared values at the core. They stress the importance of everybody incorporating the values, 'ownership' in the jargon word. Peters has as one of his key concepts that an enterprise should be 'hands-on, value-driven'. Significantly, in terms of some naive comparisons that are made between public and independent sector work, he contends that 'values are almost always stated in qualitative , rather than quantitative, terms'. 'The idea that profit is a natural by product of doing something well, not an end in itself, is also almost universal' (p.284)

Most of Peters's statements, such as a belief in being the best or a belief in the details of execution are working maxims rather than higher level value statements. Their significance lies in the fact that for these companies to be excellent, they had to get agreements amongst staff on overriding values or maxims. Within a residential home we have to move from the major value or principle statement to *practice values*: the meaning of a value statement for day to day life in terms of fairness, choice or respect for individuality. The sort of statement that would be produced is captured in a brochure about a particular school:

> Everyone, no matter what their other specific roles, takes some share in domestic cleaning, laundry, food preparation and washing up chores. Men and women share in these equally. (New Barns, 1975, quoted in Clough, 1982, p.45).

I have no doubt that it is in the working out of the detail of value statements that differences emerge between staff members. It is vital that these differences which emerge from our own past and present living arrangements are discussed and a common style agreed. One of the biggest dangers in residential work is that of staff members who undermine surreptitiously. Residential work is intrinsically different from field work in that staff have to follow each other in working with residents. This type of 'serial' work demands consistency and trust between colleagues

The knowledge required by staff includes an understanding of people and the context of their lives. Earlier chapters of this book by Peter Coleman and John Bond have examined these aspects. I want to highlight here the fact that it is probable that the people who come to live in residential homes will be those who, for whatever reason, are finding life a struggle. In part the struggle may be physical; for many it will be psychological. A knowledge of the fragility of the self of many residents will help staff to understand and to provide services.

Staff also require knowledge about mental illness in old age. It is imperative that residential workers have some understanding of the differences between confusion, depression, other mental illnesses and dementia. For example an understanding of the many reasons why a resident may be confused is vital: confused behaviour may be a consequence of shock at moving house, a bereavement, a side effect of drugs, a physical condition such as a fever or a urinary problem, or dementia. Staff must know enough to question doctors.

RESPECT FOR INDIVIDUALS

I have noted that there are institutional tendencies which lead to people being viewed as a group with common characteristics rather than as individuals. Thus, people are stereotyped as 'residents', perhaps being seen as people to be sorry for, as people who are dependent and will do nothing for themselves or as people who are always grumbling. Similar powerful forces exist in relation to groups of people who are stereotyped in society. The more dependent the older person, the more vulnerable to such stereotyping which is both about what is thought and the actions which follow. Powerful stereotyping of older people in need of services may take place in particular in relation to:

- age
- race
- sex
- disability

Readers will be familiar with equal opportunities statements: they may be pieces of paper which declare intent without having any outcome or they may affect the detail of daily living. Thought must be given to the means by which statements may be translated into practice values and action plans. Good practice in relation to equal opportunities involves challenging stereotypes, looking at the information which is provided, examining procedures by which decisions are made about who gets which services, defining the way in services are to be provided and monitoring outcome. In the end such practice is seen as the hallmark of a service which is responsive to the individual and challenges the set ways in which agencies may provide services.

A sound equal opportunities policy becomes imperative not for what some may term the soft reason of pandering to the latest fashion but from the fact that the older people who require services are vulnerable and unlikely to assert what they want. The policy should be a part of what is good practice: ensuring that the wants and needs of individuals who are provided with services and of workers are central to the life of the agency, together with ensuring that the systems and structures promote good practice in the routines of daily life.

There is not space here to highlight the myriad occasions when the consequences of stereotypes affects the services that people may receive. A few examples will have to suffice:

- men living alone are more likely to get home care than women;
- people living alone are more likely to get home care than those living with others, which may take no account of the stress on carers or the high proportions of older people of Asian origin who live with others;
- it may be assumed that people from minority ethnic groups do not want services because they wish to be cared for in their families when the reality may be that they do not know about the services or find that existing services do not match their life style;
- decisions may be taken by others which have consequences for older people because it is thought that others know best.

And so we could go on.

Providing personal services for other people is difficult, sometimes unpleasant and always demanding. We have to start by acknowledging the realities, and then plan so that people have the combination of housing and services that, within given resources, best meets what they want.

Five:

Special difficulties in adjustment

Margaret Fielden

INTRODUCTION

Throughout life we meet different challenges which are sometimes part of the expectation for the period of life which we are experiencing and sometimes are less expected and require us to make special adjustments. This chapter looks at a particular experience which may challenge people's powers of adjustment in old age.

A minority of older people are affected by senile dementia and this insidious disease presents great difficulties in adjustment both for the sufferer and for family carers. Indeed, professional carers may find some of the problems which people experience during the course of their disease very hard to handle. This chapter will look at some of the recent research which challenges traditional views of dementia. This can help us to understand better the experience of dementia sufferers and use constructive criticism to review our own approaches toward those we care for. Certain behaviours such as aggressive outbursts and wandering cause particular difficulties when trying to offer sensitive care. Here we will look at research which shows some ways of managing these problems which can be used in our care situations.

One of the challenges which can occur in later life is that of adapting to changed circumstances which limit opportunities for sexual expression, for example after the loss of a partner, where an older person or their partner is suffering from senile dementia, or in residential care. Research on this topic has opened up areas for discussion.

Our social care practices may hinder or support older people in responding to especially difficult circumstances, so throughout the chapter we will explore how the use of research evidence can help us to develop an approach to care which encourages adjustment.

THE NATURE OF DEMENTIA

The demented may not have senile dementia. The term dementia is both a description of a person's memory loss and changes in self-care and behaviour and a diagnosis of disease. Gershon and Herman (1982) suggest there may be 50 causes of dementia and that possibly 20% of these are treatable. For example a common mistake is to assume that an elderly person is suffering from senile dementia when in fact he or she is very depressed and has lost all interest in washing and cooking and appears not to remember information. This type of depression is known as pseudodementia and can be treated. Older people can become confused when they are physically ill or because their bodies are more sensitive to the effects of medication than younger people. This can result in an 'acute confusional state' which, like depression with pseudodementia, can lead to misdiagnosis. People working with older adults need to be sensitive to clues. Did this loss of memory and odd behaviour come on over days or weeks rather than the months and years expected of senile dementia? Can family or carers report events in the person's life which may have precipitated the condition? For example a series of severe losses or a physical illness or medication change may be precipitants.

Often dementia is wrongly believed to be an inevitable consequence of ageing. However, a study by Kay et al. (1964) showed that whilst the number of people suffering from dementia increases with age, only around 6% of over 65 years and 22% of over people aged over 80 years develop dementia. Because these elderly people are three times more likely to need hospital or residential care those working in these environments will see a disproportionate number of people with dementia and will need skills to manage the difficulties presented.

True senile dementia is a progressive brain disease, whether of the most common Alzheimer's type with its gradual decline of intellect and skills, multi-infarct with stepped losses or one of the rarer types. It follows a distressing pathway often with initial losses of hobbies and participation in activities, memory problems for recent events and disorientation. Later in the course of the disease the person may fail to recognise family members, lose the ability to communicate sensibly and become incontinent. In the last stages of this dreadful disease the person may become immobile and have difficulty in swallowing food. So what is the effect of this on the individual unfortunate enough to develop senile dementia?

MALIGNANT SOCIAL PSYCHOLOGY

Kitwood (1990) has looked at this question in a challenging new approach to understanding dementia and its effects on sufferer and carer. He suggests that the picture of dementia as a disease is clouded by other influences. He examines the evidence from autopsy studies of brain change in dementia and finds that the link is weak between the degree of damage to the brain and the severity of dementia the person had whilst alive. He notes the frequency of what he calls 'catastrophic decline' into dementia in some people who have been bereaved and questions whether being demented makes some sense of the confusion and threat to self-perception with the experience of great emotional pain. Many of you will have seen the difference that a trip to the pub or a show can make to a person suffering from dementia. Sometimes it appears that the symptoms of dementia decrease dramatically for the duration of the event only to return when back in the residential home or hospital ward. Tom Kitwood sees these three factors of weak links between brain damage and dementia severity, 'catastrophic decline' and variable severity of dementia in different social settings as evidence that the social experience of the person with dementia influences the severity of the disease.

So Kitwood is taking a path of understanding dementia which takes us further than a simple 'medical model' of a straightforward link between neurological impairment, that is the brain pathology, and dementia. An assumption of the medical model is that the degree of functional impairment, the level of difficulties a person experiences in the tasks of daily life is directly related to the amount of damage the disease has caused in the person's brain. The evidence Kitwood presents suggests a new model for understanding dementia where senile dementia is compounded from both neurological impairment and what Kitwood calls a 'malignant social psychology' which is a term describing the effects of a very negative social experience. Kitwood goes further. He suggests that when a person begins a dementing illness they attract to themselves this negative social experience. He goes further still in suggesting that as medical research has found links with onset of some physical illnesses, such as gastric ulcers and cancer, and stress, in physically frail older people experience of a 'malignant social psychology' may create neurological impairment.

Iif we are prepared to consider the implications of this model in our care of older adults we may be forced to question some of our practices in giving care. The 'malignant social psychology' may well be present in our efficiently run wards, residential and nursing homes and the person's own home in the unconscious and well-meaning attitudes of professional and family carers. This is not through unkindness or lack of desire to care. Kitwood stresses that his use of the word 'malignant' is to describe the effects on the person with dementia, not deliberate intent on the part of the carer. Some of the ways we may unwittingly deprive the person with dementia of what they need to continue to function as well as possible are discussed below.

Staff and certainly family caregivers frequently report that they feel under pressure and may be extremely busy, but this "busy-ness' may destroy the calm attention which will enable the dementia sufferer to be understood and encouraged to be independent. The carer may use 'tricks' to get the dementia sufferer to do what they want. The carer may not feel their schedule allows time to allow the person to do a task at their own speed, often not as well as the carer, so this opportunity to take some charge of his or her life is taken away. A person with dementia cannot think or express themselves clearly, their actions can be misinterpreted and the caregiver needs training to comprehend the effects of dementia and to enable them to empathise. Empathy is not offering sympathy or interpreting a person's attempts to communicate in your own way but trying to step into their shoes and see the world as they see it. This is not easy. For the professional carer the person with dementia will probably be unknown to you before coming into your service; for the family carer the person may have changed so much that both types of carer may 'depersonalise ' the dementia sufferer, feeling that there is not much of the person left. If so, the clues to the person's personality and experiences may then be overlooked and their human need to be understood and accepted not considered. The basis of validation therapy is that even when the person's conversation makes little sense the feelings behind what they say can receive attention and acknowledgement.

There is evidence that whilst people with dementia may be physically well cared for their emotional need to be respected as people can be ignored. Labelling a person as demented somehow separates them from society, the expectation and stigma of decline is set up. The person is no longer respected for what he or she can do or has experienced but becomes something less than normal. In a study of nurses interactions with geriatric patients in 1986, Armstrong-Esther and Browne found that the attention given to people with dementia was considerably lower than to unimpaired people. Yet many people have reported on the transformation that comes over a person with dementia when they are shown pictures or objects or hear songs, taste foods, smell household cleaning agents familiar in their younger days. Cook (1986) in a study of reminiscence groups with dementing people on hospital wards found that not only did the patients benefit, but the staff participating saw their patients in a new light; the depersonalisation was gone. Perhaps one of the greatest values of reminiscing is that it allows the older person to be seen as a person with a lifetime of experiences, to become the expert for a while and to receive attention from carers within a normal conversation rather than during the physical care which may highlight the person's disabilities.

A final factor which Kitwood suggests may prevent a carer relating to a dementia sufferer as a person can be hard to accept. Many of you may have experienced the distress following a bereavement of having people avoiding you because they find it so hard to talk to you about the death of the person you loved. This is partly through embarrassment at not finding the right words but another reason goes deeper; being reminded that death is inevitable and will affect them and their families one day can bring fear and avoidance. In the same way Kitwood suggests that the awareness that dementia could happen to us can invoke fear and an emotional distancing from the dementia sufferer so that we do not have to acknowledge that they are people like us.

This research can help us to examine our attitudes and practices to enable greater understanding of the contribution our caregiving may have on the severity of symptoms which the person with dementia presents and help sufferers to retain their sense of personhood and their skills for as long as possible.

CARE AND SUPPORT FOR SUFFERERS FROM DEMENTIA

Large numbers of old people with dementia do live alone. Arie (1991) pointed out a moral dilemma in that the level of supervision and support a person with dementia living alone requires is similar to that of young children, but statutory services put in only pockets of care for elderly dementia sufferers, and yet those leaving young children alone can be prosecuted. Many live with their spouse or children and others in some form of residential care in the private or statutory sectors. Whether the carers are family members or professional carers during the course of dementia some problems may arise which are difficult to handle. The carer may recognise the desire of the older person to find the house they once lived in or their long dead mother, but cannot practically allow that individual to leave the day lounge at that moment and perhaps this has been the third attempt to leave in ten minutes. It is not easy to bear the brunt of verbally aggressive behaviour or indeed the physical lashing out of an angry old person. Wandering was shown to cause distress to staff 50% of the time and verbal and physical abuse 90% and 92% of the time respectively in a study by Everitt et al (1991). However their study of resident behaviour and staff distress in a nursing home setting showed that staff members differed greatly in their judgement of individual residents' behaviour. Rabin et al. (1982) studied 55 family care-givers and found that 87% reported depression, fatigue and anger in reaction to the strain of constant pressure with aggressive and wandering behaviour presenting major problems. So what can be done about these types of behaviour?

These behaviour problems cause distress to professional and the 24 hour family care-givers alike and knowledge of how to manage such behaviours is extremely important, yet most family members are given no training in handling them and this can lead to a sense of hopelessness about coping. Chenoweth and Spencer (1986) found that only 16% of the 289 family carers who answered a questionnaire had been offered advice on management. Unfortunately, neither are some care staff who may have little experience of working with people with dementia and feel thrown in at the deep end when faced with a roomful of impaired people. Colerick and George (1986) showed that the support that family care-givers receive is a better predictor of future need for institutional care than the characteristics of the dementia sufferer. Care-giver training in behavioural management in an *Elderly Support Project* by Pinkston and Linsk (1984) has been shown to help family carers learn skills which prevent behavioural problems in their relative, and therefore avoid institutionalisation.

Behavioural management can be misused. It is not a block approach which can be applied to all variations of a problem. Each person's problem behaviour is particular to them and their situation and requires careful observation and recording of when the problem is occurring, where, who is around at the time, what was happening around the person, what did he or she do immediately prior to the incident and what was the immediate consequence. Each person has their own motivators which increase the chance of a behaviour occurring. It may be that a person wandering towards the doorway only gets attention from their carer at these times. If attention motivates the behaviour it becomes necessary to work out how to reduce attention on occasions of approaching the door and increase attention at other times when the person is involved in alternative activity. Only when it is possible to hypothesise about why the behaviour occurs can a behavioural programme be set up. To make it work it is necessary to record a 'baseline' measure before starting the programme; that is taking a measurement of occurrences of the behaviour usually over a two week period before making any attempt to change the person's routine or environment or carer's approach to them. Then set a time limit to test out the changes you have planned and therefore see whether the reasoning behind the programme is correct. A further period of recording the behaviour under the new 'regime' will enable an evaluation of the outcome. Decisions can then be made about whether the hypothesis about why the behaviour occurs is wrong, or alternatively whether there is a need to make the programme more sensitive to the individual's behavioural triggers and responses and change the consequences of the problem behaviour occurring.

A BEHAVIOURAL APPROACH

An example of how a behavioural approach has been used may give a clearer idea of the importance of observation and setting measurable outcome goals. Mrs S had been resident in a psychogeriatric ward for eighteen months. She was admitted via a general hospital when they were unable to handle her behaviour. Mrs S had very limited hearing and sight and did not communicate in any way. This appeared to be part of an advanced dementia. Mrs S. had a scream like a fire engine and used this very frequently. The nursing staff had not been able to relate these screams to any event and they and the other residents found them distressing. A baseline measure showed that the frequency of Mrs S's screams was 102 over a two-hour period. To make a hypothesis about why the screams occurred Mrs S. was observed very closely, one nurse suspected that she was getting grunts which resembled the word 'no' and that Mrs S's residual hearing in one ear was sufficient for communication. She devised a number of questions to put to Mrs S., some straightforward, for example 'Is it raining today?', some requiring thought 'Is the sky green?' to which Mrs S. was heard to say 'Don't be ridiculous!' A hypothesis was made that Mrs S's screaming behaviour was due to her isolation, partly through her sensory impairments but also through the malignant social environment which had developed because of assumptions that Mrs S was too severely demented to communicate. An intervention was chosen which would increase the chances of Mrs S trying to communicate in a more acceptable way by giving her opportunities to speak and rewarding her attempts with complete attention.

The intervention for Mrs S. was several short periods of time spent with her each day asking her questions about her preferences and telling her about things going on around her. An outcome measure of the screaming behaviour showed that it had stopped almost entirely. This lady had behaved in the same way for a very long time and yet after a few weeks her behaviour and her life was changed by staff prepared to challenge their own assumptions and care practice.

This lady's experience shows the importance of looking at the behaviour objectively and not seeing what the person does as an inevitable part of their dementing illness.

WANDERING BEHAVIOUR

Two studies of wandering behaviour by Hope and Fairburn (1990) and aggressive behaviour by Ware et al. (1990) have shown the need to look at the meaning of these behaviours to the dementia sufferers more closely. For example from 29 reports from community residents who cared for dementia sufferers, 'wanderers' seemed to have five types of component to their behaviour; some were excessive walkers, some trailers who needed to know where their carer was constantly, some had disturbed day/night rhythms and were active at night, some got lost on leaving their home environment and some were searching for former homes familiar to them in youth. The approach chosen to change or reduce wandering behaviour must always be tailored to the individual person and the meaning of the behaviour to them. If we observe our own behaviour for one hour I suspect that we are likely to have walked about in our environment, sometimes for a purpose but sometimes quite aimlessly picking up objects, looking at them, putting them down and moving on. Would we describe this as wandering behaviour? If we are people who enjoy exercise then could our long ambling walks be considered to be wandering behaviour? Perhaps we need to be ready to consider whether the level of walking about the person with dementia shows is appropriate and more an inconvenience to ourselves rather than real 'wandering'.

One of the biggest concerns professional and family carers express is that the person with dementia will get lost and be harmed. There is need to be certain that these fears are justified. Only where the person has been observed to leave their residence and has not been able to return without guidance may some restriction of freedom be needed. Some studies have looked at controlling wandering by making changes to the environment to stop the person going through the door without using a lock. Hussian and Brown (1987) used previous research results suggesting that people with Alzheimer's disease may have restrictions to their vision which give rise to two-dimensional patterns being perceived as three-dimensional. They found that seven of eight people with dementia in a hospital ward reduced their attempts to approach the door when eight horizontal lines of adhesive tape were stuck on the floor in front of the doorway. In a further study Hussian (1990) found that three people with Alzheimer's disease who were taught to respond to orange rectangles by associating them with food they enjoyed, but avoid blue rectangles as associated with loud noises, used this learning in their walking about their hospital ward. They reduced entry to unsafe areas when blue rectangles were placed on the walls and more frequently stayed in safe area where orange rectangles were placed.

AGGRESSIVE BEHAVIOUR.

Aggressive behaviour can be dangerous, Ware et al. (1990) found by interviewing family carers that 16 of 37 people with dementia living in the community had hit or kicked carers or thrown heavy objects. It is distressing especially to family carers to be on the receiving end and it can disrupt necessary daily tasks of washing, dressing and toileting. Most incidents of aggressive behaviour occurred when carers were involved in intimate care, or sometimes instructions given or attempts made to prevent the person doing something inappropriate provoked aggressive incidents. These types of aggressive behaviour can be seen to be related to the patterns of interaction between the carer and the dementia sufferer and can be changed by observing what triggers the behaviour and making changes in the way the carer approaches the person. We are all aware of becoming angry when we feel that we are being treated in an inappropriate way by others; our anger probably will not lead us to use physical force to make our point but we may well have our say. How much more difficult must dementia sufferers find making a reasonable response to what they perceive, rightly or wrongly, to be inappropriate behaviour towards them. In some cases the person with dementia will be right in their perception. Their aggressive behaviour may well reflect the development of Kitwood's 'malignant social psychology' where the person with dementia is treated like a child; has all decisions made for them from when he or she has lunch to future living arrangements; is tricked into doing what the carers want; is expected to do a task at the carer's pace which is greater than he or she can work at and cannot express that the things happening make him or her feel out of control of their lives and less of a person.

Research by Meddaugh (1990) supported the view that aggressive behaviour in people with dementia may be a reaction to threats to their feelings of personal freedom of choice. Observations of residents of three nursing homes in a town in the North Eastern USA showed differences in behaviour by staff toward those residents with a history of aggressive behaviour and those without. Those considered to be aggressive were given fewer choices, were approached in a less friendly manner and staff made fewer attempts to talk to them. Particularly noted were incidents where people needed physical care but were not asked or given choices about how this was carried out. Meddaugh discovered from interviewing the families of the dementia sufferers that people who had been active and 'talkers' before their illness were more likely to show aggressive behaviour. This good and bad patient behaviour was looked at by Taylor (1979) who found that people who questioned their treatment were often thought troublesome by staff who preferred passive 'good' patients. He noted that these 'bad' patients were subject to experiencing stress. This stress not only increases the likelihood of further expressions of frustration showing in aggressive behaviour but can make the person ill.

Ware et al. (1990) found that where a person with dementia was perceiving the intentions of those around them wrongly, perhaps accusing them of stealing possessions they had lost, this led to a type of 'paranoid' aggressive behaviour. This can be very distressing to family carers as can argumentative aggressive behaviour where the individual cannot be made to change his or her view of a situation. These behaviours may result from the cognitive impairment of the person with dementia where forgetfulness and losing items or the inability to think around a situation lead the person towards making faulty judgements of what is happening around him or her.

Another type of aggressive behaviour which did not appear to be related to particular incidents or to faulty perceptions was a generalised irritability. Ware et al suggest that there may be a relationship between lowered levels of a particular chemical transmitter in the brain of people with Alzheimer's disease, 5HT, which has been implicated in previous studies of aggressive behaviour. They suggest that this type of generalised irritability may respond to medication. However, on the whole most current thought on behavioural problems associated with dementia is that they are best handled by observing and recording precisely when they occur and making changes to routines or approach to the person which decrease the likelihood of the behaviour happening. This is the preferred approach because heightened sensitivity to medication in older people can increase the risk of them experiencing unpleasant side effects, and reduce their ability to respond to things happening around them.

In Ware et al.'s study some peoples' aggressive behaviour represented a change of character when they developed dementia. For others the aggressive behaviour was an extension of old ways of behaviour and a research study by Morrant and Ablog (1983) suggests that this exacerbation of traits occurs more frequently. It is difficult for the caregiver to be objective and see the behaviour as part of an illness when the person with dementia has always shown tendencies to behave this way but is now much worse.

Often it is difficult not to respond to aggressive behaviour directed towards ourselves. Interviews carried out by Ryden

(1988) in the USA showed that over a third of care-givers had felt aggressive towards the dementia sufferer and about one fifth had reacted with aggressive behaviour themselves. The problem exists and caregivers need help in understanding why the behaviour is happening and how they can best avoid it. They need to feel confident that they have skills for handling the person who shows aggressive behaviour.

Guidelines are needed for family and professional carers alike. When facing a situation known to increase the likelihood of aggressive behaviour it is important not to be confrontational or provoke the person by teasing. When there is a need for intimate care staying calm, avoiding any expression of fear, and respecting the person's personal space by not coming in too quickly, too close or from behind reduces the anxiety of the dementia sufferer; as does a clear and honest explanation of what the carer wants to do. Whatever the situation it is helpful to try to identify what is troubling the person and encourage him or her to talk about their feelings. Giving credibility to a person's right to make complaints, even if they are unintelligible, and showing awareness of the frustration he or she feels can reduce this frustration welling up into aggressive behaviour. If the approach is clearly escalating the situation walking away and trying again in a few minutes can work. The main thing the carer needs to bear in mind is that dementia sufferers have an illness which affects their understanding of their world and it is best not to take personal offence at aggressive behaviours.

SEXUAL BEHAVIOUR.

Another very sensitive area is sexual behaviour. There is no reason to consider that because someone is over fifty they are over the hill sexually. Sexual intimacy is important to many older people and special problems arise when a person suffers from dementia. Wright (1991) looked at the way that partners relate to one another when one has dementia. She found that in contrast with partners who were both well, relationships between care-givers and their partners became that of committed and dependent partners and the shared meaning in their lives together and companionship diminished. Care-givers coping strategies involved adapting to the situation and taking control in the partnership. Three of the thirty care-givers she interviewed found that an increase in the frequency of their partners' sexual advances threatened their sense of being in control.

Litz et al. (1990) interviewed husbands of women with Alzheimer's disease and the answers to their questions can help us to understand the difficulties carers experience. They found that in a partnership the unaffected person may be very distressed because their partner cannot recognise or name him or her and yet still wants sexual intimacy. The unaffected partner may feel guilty about expressing their own sexual needs in case this is taking advantage of their spouse. A person with dementia still needs displays of love and affection but because of the nature of the disease the type of sexual relationship may change with their partner unable to drop the care-giver role worrying about the effects on their spouse. When memory and concentration are severely impaired it may be impossible to maintain the sexual partnership.

Within an institutional setting sexual behaviour may be considered undesirable because of upset caused to other residents. Sometimes this upset is to staff. We need to consider whether ageist attitudes prevent us from offering privacy to people in longstanding and loving partnerships. It does not seem reasonable that the need for residential care should suddenly put a stop to the sexual intimacy of a couple who may have spent fifty years together.

In residential care staff may be put in a difficult position where they believe that an individual is vulnerable to exploitation by less impaired residents because of need for physical comfort or where a relationship is developing between two residents and staff are not convinced of both partners' awareness of their situation. Lichtenberg and Strzepek (1990) suggest guidelines regarding a person's ability to consent to a sexual relationship which develops after a person's move to residential care. Their work is based on experience of residential care and they offer examples of how their guidelines are used in practice looking at answers given to interview questions and comparing these with observations made by staff. Is the person aware of the relationship, of who their partner is or do they have false beliefs about their partner's identity, for example, falsely identifying another resident as their husband or wife? Are they able to say how far they would want the relationship to develop? Is the person's present behaviour within their lifetimes moral code and are they able to be firm in saying no to unwanted advances? If the residential arrangement is likely to be temporary, are they able to understand this and how do they foresee themselves coping with the ending of the relationship?

Some reported sexual behaviour such as self-exposure may be misinterpreted. Some individuals find clothing hard to replace properly after visiting the toilet. Another sexual behaviour takes the form of inappropriate grabs at parts of staff or residents anatomy or masturbation in a public place. First, care staff need to ensure that this behaviour is not used as a way of gaining staff attention. If the person is generally ignored but is told off for this type of behaviour the likelihood of this behaviour occurring increases. It is necessary to avoid giving attention for such behaviour but also to look for an alternative appropriate behaviour which staff can encourage and reinforce by rewarding with something the person likes, by praise or by appropriate physical contact. When the person's world of social contact is much reduced it is important to ensure that the physical closeness of a hand held, a hug offered are available. Not all want this expression of affection but it should not be denied to those who do. It is part of our humanity.

Hussian (1990) describes a behavioural approach used to change the behaviour of a man who exposed himself and masturbated on several occasions each day in lounge areas. The reinforcement chosen to change this man's behaviour was cigarettes. He was given a cigarette for each half-hour in the lounge when he did not expose himself. He was stopped and removed to his room when masturbation occurred in the lounge but there was no attempt to stop this behaviour in private. The public behaviour was completely stopped.

SUMMARY

In summary this chapter is about seeing the person with dementia as an individual with changed perceptions of what is happening around him or her, but still a person who has human needs for attention and affection and who reacts to the social world in which he or she finds themselves. It is about our responsibilities towards the individuals we care for so that we make their social world an environment which values their feelings, their rights and their choices. A social world which seeks to understand what makes them tick, why they behave in certain ways and to alter our responses to make their world less confusing and frustrating. To do this means in turn giving value to the people who care, family or professional and responding to their desire to learn how to make their caring the best they can offer.

Six:

Loss and bereavement and later life

Peter Day

INTRODUCTION

This chapter is concerned with the terminal stage of later life development and with loss and change as they affect older people. Loss is one aspect of growing older : it is a possibility throughout the life span and is inevitably encountered encountered by elderly people themselves and by those who care for them. The process of ageing can be associated with various kinds of loss - loss of paid occupation, loss of friends and relatives and physical and mental changes which may lead to disability, as we have seen in the previous chapter. We need to retain a sense of balance in that deficit and loss are only one aspect of later life. Alongside fear, anxiety and sadness about their losses older people themselves often see advantages in growing older and feel able to face up to their challenges and find ways of living as fully as possible. There are of course individual variations in ways of grieving and workers with older people need to try to understand the impact of the significant losses in their lives. In this chapter the nature of the topics is discussed first and then the research evidence about dying is reviewed. This is followed by a review of the evidence about grief and bereavement. The second part of the chapter deals with implications for older people and their carers and deals in particular with bereavement support.

The nature of the topics

It would be surprising to find anyone who feels easy about the study of death, other kinds of loss and grief. For most people these experiences are not unequivocally welcomed and this applies equally to those who are regularly involved - doctors, nurses and of course staff in residential and day care. Although there is a gradual change in attitudes and death and grief are more widely and openly discussed, we live in a society in which it remains difficult to talk about them. It is only in the last few years that some social scientists have begun to acknowledge the important part that their personal feelings play in their research and writing. Factors which it is thought have contributed to the denial of death or make us ill prepared to face it include the fact that fewer people die at home with their families and that there are generally very high expectations of health and life. Materialist values and the assessment of the worth and meaning of life in material terms mean that human contacts and relationships and non-material values are under-rated. It seems that a society which elevates materialist values creates individuals who tend to set death aside and who do not see it as part of life. By developing understanding of the way that a good deal of the confusion and anxiety about dying originates in society, staff can be helped to deal with the awkwardness and the mixed feelings dying people and those around them experience. In addition, understanding one's own attitudes and feelings about dying and grieving potentially enables one to support residents and others more effectively. This kind of insight is not fully developed merely by reading professional and other literature, powerful as these influences may be. Professional supervision is of great importance and as it provides emotional support in learning it can help staff to cope with the pain and stress of loss and grief.

In studying theoretical and empirical investigations of death, loss and grief it is important to appreciate their range. For example, work based on psycho-dynamic or psycho-analytic theories interpret individual experience of the intense distress and emotional disturbance following loss in terms of hypotheses about personal and emotional development and motivation. In dealing with processes concerning desires, wishes, fears and fantasies, they focus on the non-rational and non-logical ways in which unconscious feelings operate. In reacting to these ideas it is sometimes found that people are tempted to reject them out of hand, saying that they find them ridiculous. It is very important to scrutinise strong reactions whether they are of this kind or at the other extreme of over-dogmatic adherence to a particular theory. This is equally important in other kinds of investigation of loss and change. It is worth asking what a piece of research was aimed at. Not all investigations seek to provide interpretive data : some research seeks only to provide detailed descriptions of situations or behaviour. Some medical research is of this kind including a number of studies of bereavement. In looking at surveys of this nature it is worth checking three features in particular:

- Whether the group of people studied is typical of others in a similar situation.
- Whether the information that has been collected is accurate; for example in surveys of people's attitudes or opinions how far are they saying what they really feel or think or are they trying to impress the researcher? In studying reactions to bereavement this is a major problem.
- Whether the same results would be obtained if a study was carried out at another time or by other investigators.

To recapitulate, so far it has been noted that researchers, like anyone else, are affected by their personal feelings about research subjects. In assessing research the aims of a project and the methods employed need to be understood in relation to the subject matter. It is fallacious to regard any single theory as being the only key to complex topics and it is foolish to dismiss theories at face value. In just the same way too rigid or too literal interpretations of what a writer is thought to have said can be very misleading and can lead to harmful or unhelpful practice. An illustration of misreading results will be given in the next section.

There are problems in evaluating the results of research in bereavement. A major reason is that the conclusions from various studies are mixed and inconsistent. One difficulty in attempting to compare studies is that they have often been concerned with different populations of people from varying age brackets, geographical areas, cultures and socioeconomic strata. There is steadily growing interest in studies of individual experience and the meaning of social support for bereaved people. It is appropriate to think of the social context in which people live and die and to interpret dying and bereavement as both isolating and social events (Day, 1990).

DYING AND THE LIFE SPAN

In the context of life span development later life involves many losses and culminates in death. The older person has to adjust to decline in physical and mental capacities although later adulthood is not all physical deterioration. Older people have to sustain inevitable losses that happen to them through the death or separation of loved ones or friends. For most older people awareness of death need not inhibit the positive enjoyment of later life but can lead to greater interest in and concern for its meaning. For Erikson (1965) the task of the last stage of life is to attain 'ego integrity', an assured sense of meaning and order in one's life and the world in contrast to despair and disgust. Despair may be expressed in feelings of personal failure and regret that it is too late to redeem them. Other people may be dismissive of these feelings but opportunities to talk about them could help the older person gain a sense of perspective. Major unresolved residues of earlier life crises have repercussions on later stages. They can thus play an important part in later life, the issues being different for each individual according to past experience. Although much of the literature has avoided the subject in the past, death is central to the study of old age. Older people themselves do not seek to avoid discussion of death. The integrity of the whole of the life-span is thought to be vital to understanding old age and death. It is necessary to see people in later life in the context of their whole life history. One theory which is well known for being interpreted too literally and which was misapplied as a result is that of Kubler-Ross (1970) who identified five stages of dying. This five stage theory was interpreted in an oversimplified way by staff involved in terminal care which the author herself never intended. Many people expected dying patients to literally go through the stages as Kubler-Ross described them; and were puzzled when patients did not conform to their expectations. It is important for carers in terminal care to appreciate that a person's response to dying is far too complex to be fitted neatly into a step by step progression. Awareness that criticisms of Kubler-Ross's work were made led to alternative models being proposed (Kalish, 1978; Rodabough, 1980).

Hinton (1972) found that a considerable proportion of patients dying in hospital were observed by nursing staff to have obvious signs of anxiety taking various forms. He found ample confirmation of this and in addition a considerable number of patients described periods of distressing fear. He suggested that anxiety was not restricted to those who acknowledged that they might be dying. Often it was impossible to be sure about the reasons for fearfulness but anxiety may be generated by the emotional and social separation of a patient from family and friends at a time when comfort is most needed. On realising that they are dying, individuals often react with denial and this response may recur at various times before death. The second reaction is often anger and frustration. Anger may be expressed towards a number of people, including those caring for the dying person, of course. If their reaction is guilt, shame, grief and tears, this can increase the dying person's anger. The third common reaction is to bargain. Often individuals look for help to postpone the inevitable end of life because they realise that they have unfinished business and they need time to complete it. The fourth stage can often be depression. When anger and bargaining are felt to have failed, individuals experience a sense of loss for everything they are having to relinquish. Hinton (1972) commented on the way some people combine an awareness of impending death with extreme reluctance to die. Those who struggle in this way towards the end (or earlier in their terminal illness) experience distress and their fearful reluctance to die involves those near them. This pressure on relatives and staff can of course be very great but Hinton adds:

> Although the onlooker may find it heart rending to witness the hopeless struggle of the one who fears to die, it may not necessarily be the worst way for the patient to face his end. ..... Even the unavailing struggle may be preferable to the desolation of no hope at all (Hinton, 1972, p.103).

This response has been seen as a reaction to loss of autonomy and the ability to function normally. The individual is seen as withdrawing from social interaction as he or she prepares for death. Not everyone is able to reach the fifth stage when death is 'accepted' and it is possible to leave loved ones and to comfort them. For some people at this stage death is seen as a relief and a time for which they feel prepared.

Studies in this area which have dealt with ethnic factors are lamentably few. Cultural background and beliefs inevitably contribute to feelings and perceptions. It is an area where more research is needed and where we have to absorb and understand differences by talking to those from backgrounds different from our own. As far as death fears are concerned, it has been found in the USA that elderly black people have had more familiarity with death and are more accepting of it than elderly white people (Kalish and Reynolds, 1977). Dying people who are distressed often get enough help by sharing their grief, but in some cases psychotherapy may be helpful. A person may be troubled less about dying than about some of the consequences of being a dying person, for example by the taboo on mentioning it. It has been pointed out that a psychotherapist may help distress due to personality features such as feelings of personal failure, a burden of guilt, or by situational factors such as inability to control their lives. The part that psychotherapy can play in relieving emotional distress in terminal illness is relatively unknown but like other carers therapists need to be aware of their own reactions and feelings about dying patients (Cramond, 1970).

Religious belief is obviously relevant to many dying people. Hinton (1972) found that there was a relationship between the degree of faith and feelings of anxiety in terminal illness. Those individuals who had a firm religious faith and regularly attended a place of worship were most free of anxiety. The next most confident group were those who were straightforward in stating that they had practically no faith. There is some evidence that religious elderly people are less fearful of death than the non-religious but research results are not entirely clear on these points (Wass and Myers, 1985). Although the diversity of studies about death and dying makes it difficult to sort out and integrate results, we do have some tentative ideas from research during the last thirty years. Carers often find it difficult to talk about death. Staff in hospitals and nursing homes manage to avoid discussing it (Sudnow, 1967) and nurses respond more slowly to calls from dying patients (Bowers et al., 1975). Family contacts are often limited (Glaser and Strauss, 1968). Yet it has been found that older people are not only willing to discuss their death but actually welcome such discussion when they are given the opportunity. Young and middle aged people express more fear of death than those who are older but there are variations in death fears among older people (Kastenbaum, 1969).

ATTACHMENT, LOSS AND PERSONAL DEVELOPMENT

Psycho-analytic theory regards grief as a process of withdrawing psychic energy from the loved one, the psychological function of grieving being to separate from the dead person. It sees bereavement as re-activating anxieties and fears of early stages of development and emphasises largely unconscious feelings and emotions, personality development and family relationships. The idea that working through grief is essential for a successful outcome has been an important influence on subsequent theories. Pincus (1976) explored family relationships and reactions to loss. She said that an individual may have difficulty in coping with the death of someone if he or she had 'borrowed' his or her identity from the loved one. Feelings of anger and guilt towards the loved one and other significant figures in a person's life (for example, parents) will further hinder recovery. However most people go through grief work alone and come to terms with the problem of reinstating a lost loved person in their inner world. In psychoanalytic terms adjustment to another's death involves assimilating both the loved and hated elements of his or her personality. This adjustment is achieved through grief work which Lindemann (1944) defined as 'emancipation from the bondage to the deceased'. Going through grief work is essential to resolving grief and avoiding a pathological or atypical reaction. Lindemann (1979) said:

> This grief work has to do with the effort of reliving and working through in small quantities events which involved the now deceased person and the survivor : the tango one did together, the roles one had vis-à-vis each other, which were complementary to each other and which one would pass through day by day in the day's routine. Each item of this shared role has to be thought through, pained through if you want and gradually the question is raised. How can I do that with somebody else? And gradually the collection of activities which were put together in this unit with the person who has died can be torn asunder to be put to other people. So it can become divided among other future role partners who then become loved a little - not much perhaps at first - but become tolerable, with whom one can do things and have companionship (Lindemann, 1979, p.234).

Attachment theory provides plausible explanations for several aspects of normal and atypical grief which are otherwise difficult to understand. For example, searching for a lost attachment figure and being angry about his or her neglectful behaviour in cases of retrievable loss are functional in maintaining proximity. Whether a person reacts to loss with normal grief responses or an atypical reaction depends on earlier experience. Some vulnerable people are prone to react to loss of an attachment figure with chronic grief, for example grief which is indefinitely prolonged

(Bowlby, 1979). Further evidence has since confirmed this (Parkes and Weiss, 1983).

Attachment theory helps in understanding several aspects of normal and atypical grief which would otherwise be difficult to interpret. Bowlby (1979) regards a close bond to one or more people as being as important as food and drink. Babies have built in ways of getting their mothers to respond to them and attachment remains important throughout the life course. Individual needs for a close attachment vary at different stages and this is true of individual reactions to loss. Whether someone reacts to loss with 'normal' grief responses or an atypical reaction depends in part on their earlier experience. Adults whose childhoods were characterised by parental rejection, discontinuous parenting or threats by a parent to leave the family are often anxious and insecure. They are liable to react to loss of an attachment figure with grief which is indefinitely prolonged (Bowlby, 1979; Parkes and Weiss, 1983). Like Bowlby, Erikson (1963) saw basic trust arising through the person's close early attachments. As development proceeds the child is gradually able to tolerate greater distance from the mother. For example, by the age of three months it may be enough for her to be within sight: later still the optimum distance may be within earshot. Early childhood experience is thus seen as fundamental in emotional development and determines how children attach themselves to other people in the future and how flexible they will be in finding the optimum distance. If they do not emerge reasonably successfully from these early stages, children become rigid in attempts to find the optimum distance and their later relationships become too close, too distant or ambivalent. At any stage in development bereavement affects attachment to others. It is therefore understandable that those who have had difficulties in attachment in the past have problems in working through grief. Attachment is of overwhelming importance in the earliest years of development: Marris (1986) likens it to falling in love. The practical importance of attachment theory can be illustrated by thinking of the way grief occurs. The deepest grief is usually triggered by the loss of someone close : there is much in the situation that is a reminder of the baby's helplessness when she or he experiences separation. The mourner who weeps uncontrollably resembles a young child. At the times when the mourner gives way to these emotions, which it is necessary to express, it is important that people should be around to provide support while he or she is feeling helpless. Just as cradling a baby in your arms brings comfort, holding the old person who is sad or distressed is often valued support provided both people are comfortable about physical contact of this kind.

LOSS AND SOCIAL SUPPORT

Dying and bereavement are paradoxically isolating and social experiences and it is always important to study the influence of social and cultural factors on the process of mourning. Lopata (1979) found that grief is more rapidly resolved in societies where there is family and community support. In some countries (Japan, for example) the practice of ancestor worship enables the bereaved to keep a sense of the continued present of the dead person in the family through their religion. Buddhists believe that the spirits of the dead can be called back to the world and their mourning rituals encourage a continuing relationship with those who have died. The objective reality of loss is accepted and the disruption of the bereaved person's reality and identity is not so severe (Yamomoto et al., 1969).

Parkes and Weiss (1983) found that in cultures where the overt expression of grief is encouraged this helps counteract delayed grief responses. Ablon (1971) compared patterns of social support in Samoa and the United States and also said that grief is more rapidly resolved when social support is available. Gorer (1965) observed the marked changes in attitudes to mourning in Britain in the recent past. Religious observances for the dead are decreasing, the formality of funerals is less and there is more uncertainty about the ways of expressing grief. Gorer suggested that the lack of established ritual and of a clear structure for mourners contributes to the difficulties people have in coping with loss. It would be an over-simplification to suggest that there is a cause and effect relationship here but family and friends can help individuals recover from loss.

The bereaved person's social network is an important factor which affects the course of grief and this applies at all life stages. Grief is dealt with in different ways by different cultural groups and there is also considerable variation within them. It is important for counsellors to be sensitive about the concerns of individuals and their feelings about their religion. For people working in a multi-cultural society there is a need to be aware of different beliefs and different rituals associated with death. It is also important to note that within any cultural or religious group they will have distinct meanings for each individual. There are many ways in which the positive effects of counselling can be undermined if counsellors are unaware of complex issues of culture and race. These include inappropriate use of language, differences in non-verbal communication, prejudiced and racist attitudes and incorrect assumptions about cross-cultural counselling. Awareness of racism in society and in ourselves can enable us to work more sensitively with people of ethnic origins different from our own. A useful practical discussion of the implications of cultural variety is in Lendrum and Syme (1992).

Social support has been defined as the 'existence or availability of people on whom we can rely, people who let us know that they care about, value and love us' (Sarason et al., 1983). There is a body of evidence that the availability of social support protects individuals to some extent against the deleterious effects of stressful life events (Argyle and Henderson, 1985; Cobb, 1976; Cohen and Wills, 1985; Lynch, 1977). It may not act simply by decreasing the likelihood of encountering stressful events nor by reducing their impact but those alternatives may not be mutually exclusive. Life crises may elicit more social support from others. A number of studies have shown that bereaved people who have a high level of social support have fewer physical complaints and less depression than people who are not so well supported. Arling (1976) compared the influence of various sources of social support on the morale of elderly widows and found that contact with neighbours and friends was more influential in reducing loneliness and worry than with family members (if available).

Attachment needs do not decline with advancing age but the social isolation of elderly people is a situation from which there sometimes seems to be no escape : it may lead to entry to residential care. It is helpful to distinguish social isolation - a lack of contact with others and loneliness, which is not synonymous with solitude but is a self perceived problem. It involves a conscious lack of friendship, warmth and human contact, and is often accompanied by low self esteem. The supportive relationships available to elderly and bereaved people only exist through social networks. But these systems do not in themselves provide support : it depends on the meaning the links have for the members of the members of the systems. It cannot be assumed that because someone has many other people around them they receive more support than someone with fewer people around them. The support that an individual perceives him or herself as receiving is as significant as the actual amount of support she or he receives. Workers in residential care are familiar with the ways daily living may bring people closer together or distance them further. They are also aware, through their experience, of the way that people who are widowed, elderly and disabled are particularly vulnerable to feelings of loneliness. In grieving there is always a risk that an individual isolates him or herself from others and if this becomes extreme an extended grief reaction may result: although from a research point of view there are complicated issues in analysing the role of social support in crisis and loss and more conclusive evidence is needed about the reduction of risk, some suggestions of a practical nature can be made.

Understanding death and mourning is a personal matter but obviously cultural and religious differences have to be taken into account. When crisis or death occurs people living in an alien cultural or religious setting may feel particularly lonely and isolated. Immigrants and refugees may lack a social network and also the religious practices and possible comfort which would be available in their home land. The religious help available to all mourners needs to be considered, and not only those of different cultures: the religion of the elderly person should be noted and efforts should be made to meet their needs.

It has been thought that offering counselling to people who have experienced a stressful event in their lives may reduce distress and prevent depression occurring in vulnerable individuals. Bereavement counselling is offered on the basis of this assumption. The question remains as to whether people who are willing to be counselled are really those at risk of becoming ill with depression. Individuals who accept counselling have already recognised their need to talk about their bereavement and they constitute a self selected group who presumably believe in the value of social support in a personal crisis. Individuals who choose not to receive support may include those most at risk of breakdown. It will be evident that psycho-social support offered to dying people, their families and friends has some justification from empirical research but suggestions about how this may be provided made in the remainder of this chapter go beyond empirical research data. They draw on the accounts of bereaved people themselves and on the experience of nurses, social workers, doctors and other carers.

CARING FOR THE PERSON WHO IS DYING

Carers will usually be prepared for the person who learns that their illness is likely to be fatal to feel emotionally distressed and shocked even though this is effectively concealed. It seems obvious that if discussions are handled clumsily or insensitively the sick person will suffer considerable anxiety and depression. Abrupt and curt communication is to be avoided therefore and carers should remain available to the individual (Cameron and Parkes, 1983). Another observation worth re-iterating and constantly borne out in practice, is that some individuals are recognised as much more capable of speaking openly and honestly with dying people and of dealing with their fears. It is also likely that more staff could develop this capacity with training and support. Although many people are greatly relieved when they find that they have an opportunity to talk openly about being ill and dying there is need for caution on the part of carers. Some people react adversely to this kind of discussion and can be very distressed by references to death. A person's likely reaction may be assessed quite clearly from what they say, for example, in the way they talk about what is the matter with them. Knowledge of their ways of coping with their lives may be a valuable guide but this kind of information and carer's hunches cannot of course be infallible. Nevertheless usually it is found that a stable and warm person will probably be helped by talking about it and dealing with practical matters as well as family and friends. The people caring for the person who is dying have their own feelings about illness and death and about the reactions of the person who is dying. They may find it is helpful to have some support in sorting out which feelings are their own so that they do not confuse them with how the dying person feels. For example, one common feeling is anger towards the ill person because they are ill and dying. Seeing this anger as being aroused by his or her own fears of death does not stop the carer feeling it. But by discussing the reaction with others it becomes better understood and this helps the carer to stand back and consider how to behave towards the dying person.

Depression in elderly people is quite frequently mistaken for the early signs of senile dementia. This deep depression when people feel they are over-anxious and fearful, suffer from delusions and feel that their minds are out of control is obviously serious and potentially life threatening. Suicide rates are higher for elderly people than for any other age group. The possibility of suicide when a person decides that to continue to live is pointless is very real and a significant proportion of older people do take their own lives. In working with older people the problem is to distinguish between those who are sad and resigned and those who are actively aiming to commit suicide. To be over-aware and over-anxious about these dangers can be counter-productive : threats of suicide are often cries for help but they should be taken seriously. Threats should not be ignored. Denying the feelings of desperation that are being expressed is dangerous. A common motive in suicide is revenge and a threat is a way of showing other people how desperate an individual feels. The wish for revenge and the associated feelings of alienation and futility should be discussed if the need to punish others is to be understood.

It will be clear that the implications of work on dying are that both the needs of the individual who is dying and the feelings of those who are caring for him should be the concern of senior staff. This chapter is not intended to repeat the detailed guidance readily found elsewhere but it is probably worth remembering the tendency to neglect the obvious sometimes. Perhaps one example is sufficient. If a less experienced member of staff is involved with death the stress this causes should be recognised and support should be available. (In a similar way younger people may need time to become accustomed to the physical appearance of the bodies of older people.) The impact of the death of a resident on other residents is also very important in indicating to them the respect and care staff have for them. The need to talk openly with staff and each other if they want to do this may be a significant way to communicate caring attitudes. When death is a result of suicide it is of particular importance to recognise the anger and guilt which are experienced by other residents as well as staff and to be open to their expression.

SUPPORTING BEREAVED PEOPLE

Older people experience many stresses and grief is only one of them. It is thus frequently more diffuse than in younger age groups and often completely obscured (Cumming and Henry, 1961; Gramlich, 1968). Grief reactions are in danger of being misunderstood and misinterpreted and as mentioned before the older person may then be thought to be suffering from very different conditions (dementia, brain tumour or depression are three examples from the medical literature).

It has been pointed out above that the experience of bereavement varies greatly from one individual to another. Patterns in grieving are discernible but the degree to which individuals will experience any of the feelings involved vary according to individual personality and social contacts. Recovery time varies and older people who tend to take death badly may not complete the process. An elderly person's behaviour is sometimes puzzling until the impact of loss is appreciated. Sometimes people who are elderly keep on the move in what appears to be an aimless way or in search of a goal that cannot be defined or seems unachievable. Of course there are many reasons why someone wanders. Short term memory loss may lead someone to try to find a carer who has left them briefly and wandering may also result from boredom, loneliness, stress or physical discomfort. Walking is a way of relaxing and a way of relieving pain. Elderly people sometimes do not recognise where they live and go off in search of places they remember. They may also attempt to find people who they remember but who are unobtainable. Searching for a deceased partner, parent or child is a common reason for wandering and is a regular form of behaviour in response to separation and loss at any age. It is important to spend time in understanding the behaviour. Intervening too quickly to try to resolve the situation may be unhelpful. It is an important primary objective in working with anyone who is having to cope with grief to try to avoid additional pressures being placed on them.

One of the important issues that has not been discussed so far relates to the increasing number of older adults with a variety of disabilities who are now approaching retirement age. Some of them already in residential homes may transfer to homes for the elderly : for example older people with learning difficulties may seek to be integrated in units for their peers. As they enter the later life cycle their particular needs will require attention. Existing work on supporting people with severe learning difficulties who are bereaved is relevant in the absence of literature dealing directly with the subject (for example, Oswin, 1991). The needs of people with learning difficulties who have spent their lives in the family home and whose parents become very elderly are increasingly apparent. They may suddenly find themselves in residential care at the age of 60 years, for example, when their parents have died.

In older people depression occurs more frequently than in other age groups (Gurland, 1976) under the age of 65 years. It is usually associated with losses of various kinds, whether of status or role, or of home and friends. There is often an associated loss of purpose and meaning and an increasing feeling of loneliness. It has been found that the most socially isolated elderly people tend to be unmarried or childless people with few surviving relatives.

Their isolation tends to become a vicious circle maintained by their refusal to participate in social activities and belief that loneliness is inevitable (Townsend, 1963).

It is now generally agreed that mourning at any age can be thought of as involving four basic tasks referred to as grief work (Worden, 1983). Adjustment to loss involves great pain and effort and it is therefore appropriate to refer to it as work. If it is inhibited the grief will not be resolved. It needs to be emphasised that grief work involves a working out of complex feelings. In writing about complicated emotional processes systematically there is the danger of simplifying them too much and making the processes appear too cut and dried. People work on all the tasks at different levels throughout their bereavement. The tasks are:

- recognising the reality of the loss;
- accepting the reality of the loss;
- disengaging from what or who is lost and adjusting to an environment without them;
- building new relationships and reinvesting energy in new ways.

Anyone in contact with someone immediately after the death should recognise that the initial reaction is one of numbness and no attempt is then made to work towards recognising the loss. In the first few days or weeks the most effective way to support the bereaved is by helping with practical matters and being available when the loss is recognised (McNeill Taylor, 1983). Commonly people protect themselves from the pain of loss by denying that it has occurred, denying its meaning or denying that death is irreversible. After the death it is quite normal to hope for the return of the dead person but for most people this illusion is short lived. But the shock and denial should be seen as healthy defences against being overwhelmed by reality. The reactions are not necessary when the person reaches the point when they can confirm that the death has occurred. During this early stage support is given by coping with the varied reactions of the bereaved person through listening and understanding and not by telling individuals how they 'should' react. It is given also by indicating that death is not a taboo subject by gradually introducing talk about the death, and the funeral as well as the hopelessness, the denial and the tears. In supporting grief work on the second task, accepting the reality of the loss, carers should note whether the individual expresses the pain at being alone. They can help by continuing to encourage the recognition and acceptance that the death has taken place and by maintaining their willingness to be available to the bereaved. This means remembering what has happened and going on to look at how it affects the individual and deciding what to do about it. Individuals begin to show their acceptance of the loss when they say things like 'I am only just beginning to realise that he is dead', 'it feels as if everything has fallen in on top of me'.

If a person is unable to begin the first two tasks because the death is not accepted, it is advisable to focus on the meaning of the loss which is discussed in detail. This means encouraging the bereaved to talk about their lives with the deceased and recognise that this was in the past. There are several ways of accomplishing this, for example, by looking at photographs and mementoes, and talking about experiences like holidays that had been shared with the deceased. Basically the bereaved are asked to look at their life together before the death in detail. They can then be helped to clarify the difference between the past and the present, and to begin to experience the pain of recognition. It may also be helpful to focus on both the good and the bad sides of earlier life and on the positive and less agreeable traits of the decreased. This may enable individuals to release pent up feelings of anger, guilt and resentment, and to increase their self-esteem and more hopeful attitudes.

It is very important to encourage acceptance of the reality of loss through full involvement in what has happened. It is dangerous to deny people this involvement through seeing the body, attending the funeral and continuing to live in their own homes. Older people's needs for this kind of involvement are sometimes not understood or they are ignored because of frequent misguided ideas about their ability or inability to cope. Real anger may be directed at many people including the deceased. If it is not directed or displaced on to someone else it may be turned inward and experienced as guilt, depression and lower self-esteem. In extreme cases their feelings of anger may result in suicidal attempts and it is advisable therefore to enquire about ideas of suicide by asking 'Has it been so bad that you've thought of killing yourself?' If the individual describes ways in which he has thought of committing suicide, i.e. by explaining the method he would use it is usually thought that there is a genuine risk and that additional social work or medical help should be obtained.

The fourth task in grief work is to achieve emotional withdrawal from the deceased person and to reinvest emotional energy in new ways. The challenge of this task lies in the way the deceased has been given up but there is nothing to replace all that has been lost. Once the reality of loss has been accepted the bereaved face the meaninglessness of their lives and their loss of personal identity. This may be the most difficult period for those involved and is hindered by holding on to the past attachment. This may be due to feelings of loyalty to the deceased partner and fear of new relationships because they too might end with a loss. If at this stage the bereaved seem to be acutely sad and despairing carers and would-be helpers may feel useless and lose hope themselves. They have to try to hold on and indicate that they, at least, will be reliable. The fact that they are reliable in a period of great uncertainty and hopelessness may be of great importance to the bereaved person. They are attempting to make sense of something that appears senseless and to find new meaning in their lives. A higher proportion of older people do not resolve their grief entirely. They may suppress their grief because of their fear that to express it would be considered a sign of further weakness. Also, it may be that many unwanted changes in their lives occurring close to each other (loss of work role, loss of income, increased physical incapacity, and loss of partner) and the loss of independence and self respect, play a part. Before the individual has grieved for one loss further crises and losses have to be faced.

In seeking to support people through the process of grief work counsellors and helpers should not deny or diminish the pain that the person is feeling. Their task is to help the individual to be accepted and reassured about expressing their feelings. Much of the literature on counselling starts by emphasising a) the importance of a relaxed and comfortable setting for conversations and b) the fundamental skill of active listening (for example, Scrutton, 1989). In seeking to help people who are experiencing crises at any age, staff or voluntary workers often meet them at times when they are very emotionally upset : this is disturbing for those around including staff members. It is possible usually to find somewhere reasonably quiet and comfortable where interruptions are unlikely to occur but in hospitals and homes of course even these requirements may not always be guaranteed. The physical setting is important however and it is usually thought better for the person seeking help to sit somewhere with an undistracting view and for the interviewer or carer to sit alongside rather than facing directly. This means that the interviewee has some choice. Effective listeners develop ways of checking the speakers' motivation : how ready he or she is to talk and when they are unwilling or become tired. Having confirmed that they want to continue there are apparently simple ways of encouraging this, for example, nodding or saying 'I see'. In practice these are not simple methods but they are helpful in stressful situations. Silence is sometimes an appropriate response when someone is upset : simply holding the other person's hand or putting an arm round them may be a way of comforting them. In many cases putting an arm round another seems a natural thing to do when they are crying about a loss. It may be particularly appropriate in helping someone to let go of their feelings and to weep copiously but for some individuals body contact is not welcome and has the opposite effect. Sitting directly face to face can be inhibiting : sitting at an angle or beside another person enables both people to be more relaxed. The helper as indicated above may feel quite disturbed and tense in being with the distressed person. The implications of this simple fact are far reaching: basically where a person is angry or very upset the helper and effective listener tries to present a calm and accepting manner. This is usually found to help the situation. (It is helpful to remember that any helper can experience feelings of panic, guilt, hurt or helplessness.) It is suggested that helpers should bear in mind non-verbal messages conveyed by facial expression and bodily posture. They should try to keep reasonably still and not move suddenly, to look at the speaker and to maintain an interested expression.

CONCLUDING DISCUSSION

The subjects of this chapter, dying and grieving, involve deep personal feelings which have profound implications for theorists and researchers as well as social care staff. Those working with individuals facing death and with those who are mourning, require an awareness of their own reactions to loss and death and an understanding of how their own experiences may affect their involvement with those who are grieving. An understanding of prevalent social attitudes towards death and mourning complements personal self awareness. A range of theoretical perspectives in sociology, psychology and medicine are relevant to interpreting empirical studies of death and other forms of loss and adaptation to crises. The nature of the subjects and the vulnerability of individuals who are grieving are among the limitations on projects which can be undertaken. Dying was considered in the context of the life path (or life cycle); social and psychological support is very often valued highly by dying people and their families and friends. Grief work is important if individuals are to avoid atypical or chronic reactions. Attachment theory provides helpful indications about those people who may have atypical reactions as well as the 'normal' grieving process. Evidence that social support may protect individuals to some extent against the effects of stress was quoted. We discussed the more diffuse nature of reactions to loss in later life and some reasons that grief reactions may be misunderstood then. In general terms there are convincing reasons to see dying as a stage in the life span and not to dismiss it as negative and valueless. Stresses in the terminal stage can be coped with better if preparation is made and psychological support is available. Relatives, friends and care staff may all be part of satisfying relationships for the dying person and enable him or her to make emotional re-adjustments while receiving careful nursing and medical care.

FURTHER READING

There are several ways of approaching the complicated topics of dying and bereavement and they cannot be summarised briefly without distortion. They are subjects where contributions from academic researchers and professional people working with individuals within the terminal stage of life are complemented and enriched by the insights of poets, novelists, ministers of religion and by relatives and friends as well as dying people themselves. The range of reading available is now extensive but the following suggestions should help readers wishing to study the background to this chapter and to develop further insights into research and practice applications.

Most workers regard two publications of the Department of Social Security as basic essentials in practice. They are *What To Do After a Death* (D49) and *Help When Someone Dies* (FB29).

A book which contains much empirical data on death and mourning in social context and which is relevant to other forms of loss is by Smith (1982). Another very influential book which has a sociological perspective and which values attachment theory highly is by Marris (1986). As mentioned in the text, Bowlby's original work (1985) may be referred to and Hinton's (1972) book on dying should be of help because it is both scholarly and readable. The chapter by Hanvey in the book edited by Philpot (1989) and Scrutton's (1989) book both deal with practical issues with a sound theoretical base.

Seven:

Informal care: the research contribution

Judith Unell

INTRODUCTION

People who need help in coping with the practicalities of daily living because of age or disability have always depended primarily upon the care of family, friends and neighbours. Yet for many years the contribution of these informal carers was neglected and ignored in the design and delivery of services for dependent people. Carers remained 'the forgotten army' (Henwood and Wicks, 1984), labouring invisibly in families and neighbourhoods and often barely touched by formal services. There was an assumption, so deeply rooted that it was hardly articulated, that the continuing efforts of carers could be taken for granted and that public provision should occupy itself with meeting the needs of unsupported people.

The past decade has seen a gradual awakening among policy makers and practitioners to the scale and importance of the informal carers' contribution. Carers have come to be seen as fundamental to the government's community care strategy. Institutional solutions to problems of dependency have long since lost favour but the option of developing community care through comprehensive services devolved at local level has also foundered on the twin rocks of financial constraint and the projected explosion in the numbers of very elderly people within the population. A successful partnership with carers is now viewed as essential to a cost effective community care strategy, and the role of formal services has been recast as supplementing and extending informal care. This was, of course, a central tenet of the Griffiths Report on the future provision of community care:

> Families, friends, neighbours and other local people provide the majority of care in response to needs which they are uniquely well-placed to identify and respond to. This will be the primary means by which people are enabled to live normal lives in community settings. The proposals take as their starting point that this is as it should be, and that the first task of publicly provided services is to support and wherever possible strengthen this network of carers (Griffiths, 1988).

It remains to be seen how far this heightened sensitivity at the level of national policy will improve the lives of carers. Scepticism has been expressed about the possibility of making a real difference to carers without additional resources for the implementation of the new strategy for community care. Nonetheless, it is indisputable that informal carers have arrived on the national policy agenda and that it will be less easy to sidestep their interests and claims in the future.

Against this background, the purpose of this chapter is to make a selective examination of the contribution which research has made to understanding the informal carer. The body of relevant literature is immensely wide, encompassing studies of disabled and dependent people as well as work with a more specific focus upon carers. I have not attempted a review of the research literature, a task which has been ably performed elsewhere (Walker, 1990; Clifford, 1990). Instead my intention is to look at some of the insights gained and lessons learned in the following key areas:

- counting and describing the carers;
- looking at the relationship between formal and informal care;
- understanding the subjective experience of caring.

These areas of research activity provide the broad structure for this chapter. Wherever possible, findings relating to the informal care of elderly people are emphasised. Nonetheless it must be recognised that much research in this field focuses upon the common conditions and experiences of carers across all need groups.

COUNTING AND DESCRIBING THE CARERS

The most basic contribution of research over the past decade has been to count the number of carers within the population. Despite the commitment of both main political parties to a service strategy based upon community care, very little hard information about informal care was available until the mid-1980s. As late as 1984 it was observed that:

> No reliable data exists about the number of carers in Britain or about their characteristics and needs. Indeed this is one of the more glaring gaps in British social statistics (Henwood and Wicks, 1984).

Much of the statistical information which existed about informal care had been extrapolated from data about the needs of dependent groups, particularly the very elderly. By defining those tasks which the individual needed help in undertaking, it was possible to distinguish the contributions of different helpers, including relatives. Such information, while demonstrating the very significant role of relatives (and female kin in particular), gave little insight into the characteristics of carers or the extent of their involvement in caring (see for example, Sheldon, 1948).

Other evidence had been accumulated through surveys of women in employment. For example Hunt (1968) had found that 5% of women in the 16-64 years age group were caring for at least one elderly or infirm person within their household and 6% were providing some care for at least one such person outside the household. Later surveys tended to discover a greater burden of responsibility upon women. An OPCS survey in 1974 suggested that 13% of all women had caring responsibilities and that for those aged 40+ the proportion rose to 20% (Martin and Roberts, 1984). Hunt herself revised her earlier estimates upwards in 1978 when she indicated, on the basis of a survey of housewives, that roughly half of these women between the ages of 35 and 64 years could expect at some time to give some help to elderly or infirm persons (Hunt, 1978).

Attempts to produce a more comprehensive national picture of the numbers and characteristics of informal carers began in the early 1980s. A postal survey of carers conducted by the Equal Opportunities Commission in 1980 confirmed the unequal burden of care shouldered by women (found to comprise 75% of carers for elderly and handicapped people). It also produced figures which were projected to give a national estimate of 1.25

million people acting as informal carers in Britain (Equal Opportunities Commission, 1980).

However, the great leap forward in the supply of detailed statistical information was marked by the 1984 General Household Survey which included for the first time detailed questions about caring (Green, 1988). The finding that 14% of adults had some caring responsibilities indicated a startling figure of six million carers over the population of Great Britain as a whole. The immense scale of caring activity gave a powerful impetus to the development of lobbying on behalf of carers at national level, for example through the newly formed Carers National Association, and supported the logic of the review of community services begun by Sir Roy Griffiths in 1986.

In addition to providing a global estimate for informal caring, the GHS findings provided a basis for distinguishing between different levels or intensities of caring responsibility. It became clear that informal carers fell into different strata. Almost half of all those who identified themselves as carers devoted less than five hours a week to caring while at the core of the carer population were 1.4 million people who spent a minimum of 20 hours, including 0.7 million who carried an immensely heavy burden of care of at least 50 hours per week.

The GHS figures have not proved to be the last word on carer numbers. The more recent OPCS disability survey in 1989 produced somewhat lower estimates of the total population (3.9 informal carers and 1.1 million main helpers) (Martin et al., 1989). Differences in the definition of what constitutes care may account for some of the disparities between the two sets of findings. Also, the OPCS survey gathered information mainly from disabled adults rather than direct from carers, and thus reflects a somewhat different perspective. The provision of care for disabled children was covered by the GHS but not by the OPCS data.

Despite these differences, careful comparison of the two sets of data by Baldwin and Parker has shown significant points of convergence, notably in the size of the population of heavily committed carers.

> We are thus fairly confident in talking in terms of a population of at least 1.2 million heavily involved carers - people giving 20 to 50+ hours of care. A further 4.8 million are involved in less intense forms of care. We suspect from our reanalysis of the GHS data that women systematically under-report the number of hours they spend providing

> care, so the actual figure may be somewhat larger (Baldwin and Parker, 1991).

This analysis also showed that the most of the 'heavily involved' carers lived within the same household as the person cared for, and that the help provided by the extended family and by friends and neighbours was intermittent and limited in scale and in kind.

Pinpointing more precisely where the burden of care falls in terms of the characteristics of carers and of those they care for is a complex and difficult task. It is clear that more than three-quarters of those cared for are elderly people, most of whom fall within the vulnerable 75+ years of age group (*Education Guardian*, 1992). However, this evidence of the burden of care presented by elderly people needs to be qualified in two important ways.

First, the care needs of a large proportion of elderly people are relatively minor and straightforward - frequently confined to help with domestic tasks- and these may impose lesser demands upon their carers than the needs of younger disabled people. Second, elderly people are not simply at the receiving end of informal care but very active in providing it for all dependent groups other than children. In particular, the carers of elderly people are frequently spouses of similar age. The stresses of caring are likely to bear particularly heavily upon these elderly carers who may well have health problems of their own and who will have few opportunities to escape from the caring situation, for example through undertaking paid employment (Peace, 1986).

The gender bias within the population of carers has been the subject of much comment. It has been widely accepted that the provision of informal care has in practice been women's work:

> In the field of social care the terms 'community' and 'family' have for too long masked the fact that it is female kin who carry out the bulk of caring and tending (Qureshi and Walker, 1986).

Successive studies have demonstrated the destructive impact of caring upon women's personal well-being, wider family relationships and participation in the labour market. A predicament which has been widely reported is that of the woman with children still living at home who is torn between meeting their needs and those of an elderly dependent relative (for example, Ungerson, 1987).

The recent survey evidence has produced rather more equivocal findings on the subject of sexual inequality in caring. Indeed the GHS survey found that similar proportions of men and women were involved in caring, although the absolute number of female carers was greater because of the bias towards women at the older end of the population. Closer analysis has suggested that the considerable majority of male carers are elderly spouses. If there is no spouse to provide care, then it would appear that caring responsibilities are devolved to children, primarily daughters and daughters-in-law (Baldwin and Parker, 1991).

The preponderance of women as carers of physically and mentally frail elderly people is well-documented. Indeed Levin et al. (1989) have suggested that women account for 70% of carers for this group. Thus it is clear that women are disproportionately involved at the 'heavy end' of caring. Even at lower levels of dependency, women are more likely than men to be involved in personal care such as dressing, bathing and toileting. Men are primarily providers of physical and practical help such as help with getting out of bed, walking and completing tasks around the home.

The thrust of the research evidence therefore suggests that women are expected to take on more complex and challenging caring commitments than their male counterparts and that these involve women in a greater degree of conflict between their role as carer and other family responsibilities. Observers have not been slow to point out that this burden of care for women is likely to be increased by current policies which identify informal carers as the front line of community care and by the recession in the labour market which offers women fewer choices in terms of paid employment.

Available data about labour market participation by women carers of elderly people are difficult to interpret. Small-scale studies have repeatedly suggested that the carers - mainly women - of frail elderly people have made considerable changes to their working lives, including giving up work altogether, in order to continue to care (Martin and Roberts, 1984). However, the findings of the 1985 GHS survey suggested that working-age carers of elderly people were more likely than any other group of carers to be in some form of paid employment. Parker and Baldwin's reanalysis also showed that female carers in this category were as likely to be in work as female non-carers of the same age (Baldwin and Parker, 1991).

However, reduced levels of labour market participation were evident for carers of both sexes who were called upon to provide more intensive, personal forms of care. Given that such care usually falls to women and given the projections of increasing numbers of very frail elderly in need of this level of support, it might be expected that a significant and increasing proportion of women will be finding difficulty in reconciling their caring and working commitments.

This leads directly to the important question about whether the supply of informal carers in the future will be sufficient to meet the needs of elderly people, particularly the very old and frail whose numbers are increasing rapidly compared to the elderly population as a whole. Projections of the size and dependency profile of the elderly population may be the root of this concern but they are linked to other factors which threaten to disrupt the infrastructure of informal care. These are principally the shrinking numbers of potential carers, particularly women, in the 45 - 59 years of age group; the increasing tendency among women of this age to seek paid employment; patterns of geographical mobility which affect the capacity of families to care for elderly relatives; and the increasing incidence of family breakdown which may disturb existing patterns of support and care across the generations.

Each of these trends provides a major area of study in its own right in terms of its impact upon informal care. Taken together they do strongly suggest that the need for care by elderly people is increasing faster than the supply of family carers. Sensible voices have been raised against alarmism, pointing out, for example, that much of the so-called dependency among the elderly is the result of the negative social conditions and expectations which surround old age in our society (see for example, Wells and Freer, 1988). While socially constructed dependency of this kind is amenable to intervention and improvement, there nonetheless remains a large and growing number of mentally and physically frail old people who will require committed and intensive support if they are to remain in the community. It would be unrealistic and unjust to plan on the assumption that informal carers can continue to shoulder such a responsibility alone with occasional help from outside. At the same time research has shown the complexities and difficulties of building a working partnership between informal carers and formal services.

THE RELATIONSHIP BETWEEN FORMAL AND INFORMAL CARE

An important and interesting stream of research has concerned itself with the distinctive features and organising principles of formal and informal care. Such work has provided an important theoretical perspective on the problems of organising formal services in a manner which supports but does not exploit the informal carer.

The seminal work in this area is that of Abrams. His contribution was to change the conception of formal and informal care as points along the same spectrum of care-giving. He asserted that these were instead separate systems which did not co-exist comfortably. Indeed he implied that formal services posed a threat to organic systems of informal care (Abrams, 1977; 1978).

According to Abrams, the key difference between the two systems was that while the delivery of formal care was determined by standardised criteria of need, the giving of informal care was based upon the recognition of obligation and reciprocity within a social relationship. A consequence which flowed from this difference was that informal care could not be explicitly defined or prescribed; instead it developed out of the relationship between the carer and recipient. It was necessarily diffuse and idiosyncratic whereas the delivery of formal services depended upon specific, prescribed methods and outcomes.

Abrams recognised advantages and disadvantages in both systems. The bureaucratic framework surrounding formal services brought rigidity, delay and professional domination; on the other hand, such agencies dispensed valued resources in a relatively rational and even-handed manner. Informal care was patchy and unpredictable in its impact with no mechanism for ensuring that care was given to those most in need or that the requirements of actual recipients were fully met. However, people were cared for because they mattered to the carer rather than because they fitted within an agency remit. This created important *intrinsic benefits* within the caring relationship in terms of emotional rewards for both parties which, in Abrams view, were the crowning virtue of informal care. Given the choice, he argued, people in need would prefer to receive services from those close to them rather than from formal care providers.

It is important to remember that while Abrams recognised the value of informal care, he did not exaggerate its capacity. In particular, he sought to demolish the myth of an active, caring local community. In his view, informal care within a modern industrial society could exist only within the family or within moral communities such as churches. This has indeed been the conclusion of successive studies of informal care and is also the finding of the GHS and OPCS surveys discussed earlier which indicate that the contribution of neighbours and friends is peripheral when compared to that of children and spouses.

Abrams work thus provided a valuable corrective to an over-simplified and romantic view of community care. It also challenged the notion that the provision of care simply requires the coordination of the efforts of formal and informal carers to achieve a common goal. It is clear that informal care will not submit to this kind of discipline or organisation.

Nonetheless, the argument about the 'superiority' of informal care was to prove a two-edged sword. On the one hand, it accorded recognition to the value of the work of informal carers'; on the other, it gave a superficial legitimacy to the government's claim in the early 1980s that spending on public provision of community care should be checked in order not to undermine community self help:

> Whatever level of public expenditure proves practicable, and however it is distributed, the primary sources of support and care for elderly people are informal and voluntary. These spring from personal ties of kinship, friendship and neighbourhood. They are irreplaceable. It is the role of public authorities to sustain and, where necessary, develop - but never to displace such support and care (DHSS, 1981)

The notion of public authorities displacing their role is likely, at best, to provoke wry amusement among carers. A large body of research evidence suggests that carers have been systematically starved of resources by formal services which have operated according to a crisis model of service provision, providing help only when other care resources have broken down. In 1976 Moroney pointed out the pitiful level of support for families coping with a frail elderly or mentally handicapped dependent. He concluded that the lion's share of resources for these groups was being consumed by residential care services which catered only for a small minority of people in need, leaving an inadequate domiciliary service targeted primarily at those without family support (Moroney, 1976).

This imbalance between residential care and community services was exacerbated during the following decade as financial restraint bit into the budgets of social services departments and a massive expansion in private residential care, particularly for the frail elderly, was fuelled by social security payments. This was the situation which Sir Roy Griffiths and his advisers addressed in their review of community care policy (Griffiths, 1988).

What has happened since is a planning process geared towards a strategic realignment of services with the primary objective of enabling as many dependent people as possible to remain in their own homes. At the time of writing, community care plans are being finalised across the country, in many cases incorporating for the first time in public policy planning the expressed views and needs of informal carers. Nonetheless, Abrams' doubts and questions remain pertinent. Given that they operate within separate spheres, how is the boundary between formal and informal care to be negotiated in the provision of services?

Perhaps the key issue is how to make services available which relieve the burden of the carer without diminishing the well-being of the person cared for. As Qureshi and Walker rightly point out in relation to services for the elderly, an approach to service-provision which promotes the interests of one partner in the informal caring relationship at the expense of the other, is likely to bring destructive and unacceptable results for both parties (Qureshi and Walker, 1986). For this reason they dismiss the arguments of some feminist writers in this area, notably Finch (1984), that residential care should take over the role of care provided by female kin, pointing to their own evidence from a research study of informal caring in Sheffield that :

> 'Overwhelmingly, both elderly people and carers want the disabled elderly person to continue to live in familiar surroundings (Qureshi and Walker, 1986).

If the emotional satisfaction of being cared about is essential to the well-being of the elderly dependent person, can this feeling be reproduced within a relationship with a care provider who has a formal status? Several researchers have suggested that this does indeed happen and may be particularly likely when the provider is a volunteer who may be readily assimilated into a quasi-informal role. For example, a study of volunteer visitors to the elderly showed that the formalised nature of the relationship was significant only at the outset and that personal interest and friendship often grew between visitor and visited (Seyd et al., 1983).

Similar findings have been reported in relation to home helps or care assistants (Sinclair et al., 1984). It is clear that many develop a commitment to particular clients which extends beyond the boundaries of their formal duties. This may involve, for example, visits outside working hours, performing extra tasks, or inviting the elderly person to their own homes. However, as Qureshi points out, this engagement with a client can only happen voluntarily and selectively; it cannot be required or expected within the terms of the job without losing its meaning to both parties (Qureshi, 1990). Informal social rewards depend upon a person-to-person exchange which transcends the relationship of worker and client. Thus although formal services may in some circumstances offer qualitative benefits similar to those provided by informal care, it is clear that they cannot be counted upon to do so.

An alternative strategy might be to try to stimulate the supply of carers artificially so that caring tasks are more evenly and consistently distributed, while at the same time guaranteeing a personal service to the recipient of care. The most obvious means of doing so is by offering payments to carers for services rendered. There have been some examples in the UK of paid 'good neighbour' schemes for the elderly based upon this idea; so far, however, there have been no comparable initiatives targeted at family carers. Financial payments to carers are limited to the social security system and are designed to provide a standardised, minimal level of support.

Although financial rewards for family carers would be welcome in their own right as a source of help and recognition, available research does not promise a significant impact upon the numbers of people preparing to take on a caring role.

The evidence overwhelmingly suggests that carers do not sit down and calculate the costs and rewards of caring before they become involved. In the first place, people do not generally become carers as a matter of deliberate and conscious choice. Characteristically they 'drift' or 'slip' into a caring role within an existing relationship because of changing conditions. Second, as Qureshi describes in relation to a study of informal carers for the elderly in Sheffield, there is a well-defined hierarchy of obligation within the kin network which is highly effective in assigning caring responsibilities to particular individuals (Qureshi, 1990). People become carers because of a sense of duty often combined with a feeling that 'there's no-one else to do it' and a sense of personal debt towards the elderly person. It is unlikely that external incentives would significantly modify this informal system. Moreover, the notion of an exchange of labour for money cuts across the dynamic of the caring relationship in which labour is given because of feelings of love and obligation. Although financial exchanges may feature within this relationship, they have no formal, contractual basis.

In any case it is unwise to assume that there is an untapped supply of family carers which could be mobilised if only the proper incentives were offered. The demographic and economic trends referred to earlier suggest instead a diminishing number of people able to undertake the care of elderly people within their own families. Furthermore, most studies of informal care reveal existing family carers working up to and beyond their personal limits.

If the numbers of committed family carers cannot be increased through artificial means, it is at least possible that formal services may be organised so as to reproduce some of the benefits of informal care. Several schemes have now been undertaken and evaluated which aim to support frail elderly people in the community by offering maximum flexibility, continuity and choice of services. Perhaps the best known is the Kent Community Care Scheme, later replicated in other areas. The evaluations of the Kent Scheme and similar initiatives by the Personal Social Services Research Unit at the University of Kent have offered valuable insights into the impact of this approach upon the elderly person and upon existing carers.

The key elements in the Kent model are individual case management by experienced local authority social workers combined with decentralisation of care budgets, enabling resources to be spent at a local level both on existing services and on additional help to fill gaps. Agreements are made with voluntary and private bodies and with individual members of the community to provide services or to perform specific tasks in return for payment. Such schemes have achieved good results in terms of enabling the elderly person to remain within the community for longer periods. However, their impact upon carers has been equivocal. Reviewing the findings relating to the Kent Scheme and to a similar scheme in Gateshead, Walker notes that although the 'subjective burden' of existing carers was found to be eased by the intervention, there was no reduction in the amount of time they devoted to caring and no significant amelioration of the practical and financial problems they faced. She suggests that the benefits to carers might have been more substantial if the intervention had taken place at an earlier stage of the cared-for person's dependency (Walker, 1990).

It is evident that schemes which aim to provide support by complementing informal care must address the separate needs of carer and cared for if they are to bring real benefits to both parties. Existing schemes, like more mainstream statutory provision, have taken the needs of the cared for person as their principal focus, often treating carers as a resource and discounting the costs to them of continuing to care.

A different approach is to create services whose primary aim is to meet the needs of the carer. There are now many examples of services, flexible residential respite care, Crossroads care attendant schemes, family foster care and carer support groups. Walker points out that although such initiatives are generally set up according to the most sympathetic and carer-centred ideas, they are rarely subject to rigorous appraisal and their impact upon the well-being of carers is therefore difficult to assess. Many are ad hoc developments, often set up in areas with an under-provision of mainstream services. In such circumstances it is difficult to judge whether the reported benefits of an intervention are different from or greater than would result from an adequate level of conventional provision (Walker, 1990).

Thus formal provision can be seen to fall into three broad groupings. At the core are mainstream services which provide the bulk of support for dependent people within the community but whose effectiveness in terms of carer support has been blighted by divisions between the provider agencies, by an inappropriate level of worker specialisation at the front line and by an informal rationing system which discriminates against carers. Next there is a limited number of community care schemes which mobilise a wide range of formal and informal resources and offer an integrated, non-specialised service to dependent people; such schemes may bring incidental benefits to carers but this is not their primary objective. Finally, there is a scattering of initiatives focused upon the provision of carer support.

What exists, therefore, with some imaginative exceptions, is a system of formal service provision which is poorly organised for meeting carers' needs. Changes will be needed if the shift in public policy towards supporting and relieving informal carers is to be translated into effective provision. Research has helped to define what these changes should be.

First, the policy of withholding practical help from elderly persons with carers must be abandoned. As Levin et al. (1983) have pointed out, the concentration of these resources upon people living alone is short-sighted and misguided:

> In this study, as in others, we found that home helps went predominantly to those who lived alone. A consequence of this policy was that home helps served elderly persons who were in many ways least difficult to manage (Levin et al., 1983).

The important preventive effects of providing practical help to carers before they reached the point of total exhaustion were also highlighted by this study.

In reviewing policies for the allocation of resources, it will also be necessary to question some beliefs about informal care which have lain undisturbed in the minds of service planners since Abrams' research. For example, the assumption that elderly people will prefer care which is provided by those close to them because of the emotional rewards which it brings needs to be qualified by the recognition that many welcome additional help as a source of relief for their carers and, furthermore, that they are able to view such services in purely instrumental terms.

Similarly, the belief that carers prefer to take on the primary responsibility for caring must be set against the evidence from several studies that most say they would have welcomed help if only it had been offered. It is clear that both carers and those they care for see formal services as a needed supplement to informal care. There is evidence of strong support for this view among the population in general. A study of public preferences for the care of dependency groups undertaken by West et al. (1984) indicated only limited support for informal care as the preferred option without extensive professional involvement:

> What the public want is not care *by* the community, nor residential care, except in specific circumstances, but a range of community based services which best serves the interests of dependency groups and alleviates the burden of carers (West et al., 1984).

The second change which is needed is the creation of a more flexible and versatile model of service delivery along the lines pioneered by the Kent Community Care Scheme and similar initiatives but taking more fully into account the carer's separate needs. The difficulty in achieving this flexibility outside flagship schemes is that it runs counter to the trend within health and social services towards increasing professionalisation and specialisation. As Waerness (1990) points out, any moves towards despecialisation in the provision of services are likely to encounter resistance from professional organisations and open up a latent conflict of interest between service providers and consumers.

Nonetheless, if the objective is to design a system of provision which supports and enhances the caring relationship, the logic of moving towards a more integrated and flexible service system is irresistible. This point was made strikingly by Bayley (1973), in his study of mentally handicapped people and their families when he demonstrated that the efforts of sustaining the daily grind of caring left little energy in reserve for adapting to the routines of statutory service providers. Unless the services learned to do the adapting, he concluded, they would be of little benefit to dependent people and their families. Ten years later, Meredith and Lewis made a similar observation that carers require elaborate routines in order to survive, and concluded:

> In this sense informal care is extraordinarily inflexible and it is the formal support that must be flexible enough to meet individual need (Lewis and Meredith, 1988).

A third change should be the development of a more proactive approach in identifying informal carers and offering support. Existing support systems for carers depend largely upon self-referral. However, research has shown that carers find it difficult to come forward. This is partly because of the widespread lack of information about available services but also, as discussed below, because carers have complex and ambivalent feelings about their responsibility to care.

Publicity which helps people to recognise themselves as carers and which informs them about the help on offer is indispensable to a positive outreach strategy. Even more important, however, is to make better use of existing entry points to formal services, notably general practitioners, as a means of identifying vulnerable elderly people and their carers. At present there appears to be widespread under-identification. In particular, research has shown that general practitioners are prone to disregard mild social and behavioural problems among their elderly patients, with the result that opportunities are lost for providing assessment and support at an early stage before the carer becomes exhausted (Levin et al., 1983).

To sum up, research suggests that, formal services must be committed to certain key principles if they are to provide effective help for dependent elderly people and their carers. These are that:

- there should be no discrimination against carer households in the provision of support;
- that the separate needs of the carer and the dependent person should be considered;
- that services should be integrated and flexible at the point of delivery;
- that services should take a positive and active approach towards the sharing of care as soon as possible after caring has begun.

These principles provide a framework for shared care within which the individual needs and preferences of carers and dependent elderly people may be negotiated.

THE SUBJECTIVE EXPERIENCE OF CARING

The subjective experience of informal care has been a lively research issue. Most studies have focused upon the carer and have attempted to measure the impact of caring in terms of personal and psychological costs. A different strand of research has taken a more dynamic, interactive view of informal care in which the experience of the carer is viewed against the changing nature of the caring task and relationship with the person cared for.

Studies of carer functioning have usually adopted a clinical methodology in which the psychological and social well-being of subjects are measured using standardised instruments and compared with a matched control group. The findings of such studies have almost universally shown raised levels of stress and morbidity among carers. For example, a study by Jones and Vetter of 256 carers of elderly dependent people found that levels of anxiety and depression were considerably higher than within the normal population. It also found widespread distress among carers at the curtailment of their social lives (Jones and Vetter, 1984). A smaller and more in-depth study of carers of confused elderly people at home found very high levels of reported distress, with one-third reporting a sufficient number of symptoms of acute distress as to suggest a need for psychiatric attention (Levin et al.). Levels of strain were found to be strongly associated with admission of the dependent elderly person to residential care within the following year. Once again, very high levels of psychiatric distress were discovered in a study of a Scottish day hospital (Gilleard et al., 1984).

Evidence about the impact upon the physical health of carers of elderly people is more equivocal, largely because many carers are themselves elderly, with the disabilities and problems commonly associated with old age. However, as Walker points out:

> Arguing about whether the physical burdens of caring cause physical health problems is perhaps a canard. Carers undoubtedly do experience a great deal of physical exertion in their daily living, far above that experienced by other people, which does appear to restrict their lives in many ways. Moreover, physical ill-health does seem to be associated with reduced duration of informal care (Walker, 1990).

Some researchers have sought to counterbalance the negative evidence about the impact upon carers by identifying benefits and rewards but these look fleeting and insubstantial when set against the overwhelming evidence of the toll taken by the daily grind of caring. At the same time it is clear that most carers have a strong commitment to their role and wish to continue caring even at considerable cost to themselves. The motivation to care cannot therefore be understood in terms of a rational calculation of personal costs and benefits; as noted earlier, it is embedded within the relationship with the person cared for.

The subjective quality and dynamics of this relationship have received little research attention when compared with the 'objective' measurement of carer distress. In particular there is little understanding of how the caring relationship is perceived by the person cared for. However, several studies have now explored the relationship from the carer's perspective and developed an understanding about how patterns of caring and dependency unfold over time.

In probably the majority of caring relationships, the role of carer is assumed gradually and almost unconsciously. It has been widely reported that even people with quite extensive caring responsibilities may have difficulty in perceiving themselves as carers. This is because the caring role is seen as a 'natural extension' of the mutual care that is intrinsic to family relationships. The phenomenon of 'just slipping into' the carer role seems to be most likely when the partners in the relationship are co-resident, either as spouses or as child (usually daughter) and parent. However, it would appear that carers in general take their responsibilities for granted. Qureshi (1990) found that the (predominantly female) carers in the Sheffield study referred to earlier seemed to be 'taken aback' when asked why they provided care:

> Where explanations were offered they tended to be either simple statements of the family relationship...or, alternatively, explanations of why some other member of the family did not help...It seemed that there was an implicit set of expectations about who should provide routine assistance to elderly people, and that actions in conformity with these expectations were so obvious as not to require explanation. Only where the carer was 'unexpected', as in the case of the niece, was any explanation necessary.

Lewis and Meredith, in their study of single daughters caring for elderly mothers, make similar observations about the power exercised by the 'injunction to care' upon these women (Lewis and Meredith, 1988). Whether or not a conscious choice had been made to care, the women felt that it was right for them to be doing so. These feelings seem to echo the observations made by feminist writers on informal care, notably Gilligan (1982) and Graham (1983), that the obligation to care is deeply internalised within the female psyche to the extent that it has become a component of feminine identity. Thus women tend to judge themselves by their capacity to provide care and feel guilt if they see themselves as failing to do so.

The unquestioning assumption of caring responsibilities does not of course mean that carers adjust happily and easily to their role. On the contrary, as the studies of carers' psychological health indicate, caring is the source of widespread distress. A great deal of qualitative evidence confirms that the caring role is the focus of emotional conflict as carers try to balance the obligation to care with other responsibilities and their need for personal autonomy. This conflict tends to be greater for women, partly because of their profound commitment to the notion of providing care, but also because they tend to take on more complex and demanding caring tasks than their male counterparts and receive less support in doing so. Several studies have suggested that role conflict is also greater for adult children carers than for spouses since the former are more likely to be subject to competing demands on their time and to be required to make painful adjustments to their own lives in order to continue to care, (for example Bowling, 1984).

Thus the subjective experience of caring is likely to differ according to the gender of the carer, the carer's health, and the nature of the relationship between carer and cared for. These factors may perhaps be considered as constants within the caring relationship. In addition there are more dynamic elements which arise from the particular caring situation and which have a profound effect upon the carer's subjective burden.

Common sources of carer strain indicated by several studies are difficult behaviour on the part of the dependent elderly person, a loss of closeness between carer and cared for once the caring relationship has begun, and restrictions upon the freedom of movement and social contacts of the carer. These interact in complex ways with the contextual elements in the caring situation so that, for example, they will tend to have maximum effect when the carer is co-resident with the cared for, when the carer is female and when she is in poor health herself (Sinclair, 1990).

This kind of analysis is a valuable aid to assessment. It shifts the focus of attention from the condition of the dependent elderly person towards the caring relationship. By identifying likely sources of carer strain, it provides a more sophisticated understanding of how support services might be best applied. A possible drawback is that it gives rather a static 'snapshot' view of the caring relationship. In reality, this relationship is dynamic and unstable. The changing condition of the person cared for alters the objective circumstances and subjective experience of the carer. Even during a stable period, the carer's experience will be affected by her *perception* and *expectations* of how the commitment to care will change over time.

In his insightful analysis of the concept of caring or 'tending' Parker (1981) recognises the significance of locating the caring relationship within a time frame. He identifies four dimensions of tending which are most important in differentiating one caring experience from another and which thus help to explain the varied responses of carers. According to this classification, the *intensity* of the support required, ranging from perhaps 24-hour care to weekly assistance, and the *complexity* of the caring task, in terms of the special skills required, interact with the expected *duration* of care and the *prognosis* as to whether more or less care is likely to be required as time passes.

An understanding of the dynamics of the caring relationship is also central to an important study undertaken by Meredith and Lewis. From their in-depth retrospective interviews with adult carer daughters of elderly mothers, they were able to identify three broad stages of caring as part of a *caring sequence*. These were semi-care, part-time care and full care. Most of the daughter carers progressed through all three stages (Lewis and Meredith, 1988).

At the semi-care stage, the daughters felt considerable disquiet about, and responsibility for their mothers even though the latter did not overtly require care. At this stage both mother and daughter were able to retain independent friendships and contacts. A sudden event such as a stroke or a more gradual but noticeable deterioration in the mother's physical or mental condition would trigger the next stage of part-time full care in which the carer assumed full caring responsibilities but tried simultaneously to maintain an independent life within and outside the home, sometimes including paid work. At the final stage of full care the carer capitulated to the demands of caring to the exclusion of other commitments.

Critical observations from this study were that the quality of the caring relationship appeared to deteriorate along with the growing dependency of the elderly person and that it also became more exclusive as outside interests fell away and the carer assumed greater responsibility for personal and physical care. Most daughters perceived the relationship with their mothers as problematic once the caring sequence had begun even in those cases where a good rapport had existed up to that point. Paradoxically, it became more difficult for the carers to obtain outside help once the relationship had deteriorated to the point where they badly needed a buffer against stress. This was partly because of a lack of information about services and, in some cases, because of misgivings about the suitability of the help that was on offer. But beyond these practical obstacles lay a profound ambivalence about calling for help which was in turn rooted in a sense of loyalty to the person cared for and feelings of guilt about their own inability to cope.

Qualitative research evidence of this kind contains vital lessons for service planners. First of all it demonstrates the complexity of emotions and attitudes within the caring relationship. A professional assessment of need is clearly inadequate as a basis of action if it disregards their feelings about each other and about outside sources of help. Second, it shows how the stresses and demands upon the carer change as the caring sequence unfolds. Once again, intervention needs to be sensitive to this dynamic. Thus in addition to providing help which is relevant to needs at the point of assessment, service planners might think about timing their intervention so as to prevent deterioration in the caring relationship. This might, for example, involve providing extra support for carers whose network of friendships and interests is still intact rather than waiting until these resources have collapsed.

CONCLUSIONS.

Research into informal care has illuminated the scale of the contribution made by carers and the considerable personal and social costs which this entails. It does not invite complacency about social policies which assume that informal care is capable of extending itself to cope with a growing population of frail and confused elderly people. Demographic and social factors indicate that at a time when the caring task is becoming more difficult, the supply of carers capable and willing to take it on is diminishing.

In this context there is a need for better ways to connect the systems of formal and informal care. This will require the reversal of a long record of failure on the part of formal services to recognise the importance of sharing the burden of care and to offer appropriate support. Research has demonstrated the need for maximum flexibility and integration of service delivery, and the importance of an active and positive attitude in making help available. A policy framework is now in position to facilitate such an approach but obstacles remain in the form of professional attitudes which promote increasing differentiation and specialisation of services, and, most crucially, in chronic resource constraints.

Above all it is important to recognise that the function of formal services is not, as has been assumed for so long simply to plug gaps in the care provided by families. To make community care effective, formal services must give the highest priority to sustaining and relieving informal carers. In some cases this will mean allowing individuals to stop caring.

Finally, research has shown that informal care grows out of a social relationship which continues to develop and change during the caring process. It has a strong emotional content. This relationship must be understood and respected by those offering help from outside. Otherwise help will be rejected and the isolation so commonly experienced by informal carers will be reinforced.

Eight:

The contributions and needs of formal or paid 'carers'

Chris Payne

INTRODUCTION.

The purpose of this chapter is to examine the contributions made by 'formal' or 'paid' carers to the quality of service provision for older people, and to indicate how research can guide and assist them in their work. By 'paid' carers we mean people, who are employed for a wage or salary by public, voluntary or private agencies to provide care services to older people in their own homes and in institutional settings such as day centres and residential homes.

CONTRIBUTIONS OF RESEARCH.

Research into both domiciliary and residential social care is now extensive, as exemplified by the number of reviews of studies and findings currently available (e.g. Sinclair, 1988a; National Institute for Social Work (NISW) Practice and Development Exchange, 1988; Sinclair et al., 1990; see also Goldberg and Connolly, 1982). Nevertheless it is difficult to identify specific research studies that are directly relevant to the practice and training needs of paid carers and their supervisors and managers. Generally the areas of research that have implications for care practice, organisation and management, and training include:

- the needs of older people for services, including applications for and admission to residential care;

- the form, content and intensity of the service provision itself, in relation to identified needs and its effectiveness in meeting those needs (for managers certainly there is the burning issue of how to distribute resources most equitably and effectively and the establishment of priorities);
- the process of providing and receiving services, including, for example, the differential use made of day, respite and short stay residential care;
- the process of admission to residential care as a possible permanent move;
- the quality of residential life and how this can be improved;
- the views, attitudes and expectations of the older people themselves as 'consumers'.

Such studies are referred to throughout this chapter.

WHO ARE THE 'PAID' CARERS?

Taking into account the numbers of home carers, 'home helps', staff in residential and day services employed by local authorities, private and voluntary sectors, and others employed on special schemes, for example Youth Employment and Employment Training Schemes , 'caring' is now one of our biggest 'industries'. Home carers and care assistants in day and residential services clearly make up the majority of the workforce of local authority social services departments. As Clough (1986, p.83) comments, 'there can be no dispute with a statement that staffing consumes the major proportion of spending on residential care.' However it is almost impossible to calculate accurately the total size of this essential but undervalued workforce, without whose efforts the whole service system would collapse.

The Wagner Report (Wagner, 1988, p.71) includes numbers of residential staff taken from a 1987 workforce survey, with a total of 238,900. However, these figures, which aggregate direct service, management and supervisory, and domestic and ancillary staff, refer to all residential services staff including those working with children. They do not include home helps. A 1991 Workforce Analysis gives the number of manual staff (home helps and residential care assistants) as 150,000 and 'officer' staff in residential, day and domiciliary services as 54,000 (LGMB, 1991). But these would include staff employed to work with other than older people.

As a 'guestimate' the total numbers of people paid to care for older people in one capacity or another must be near or in excess of 500,000. However, it is virtually impossible to obtain accurate statistics for services as a whole; it needing to be noted that private homes are now the major providers of residential services. Neither their staffing patterns nor levels are directly comparable with local authorities.

For the private and voluntary sectors to date very little research into staffing composition, patterns of employment and deployment, methods of recruitment and selection, reasons for staying or leaving has been attempted. From the limited information available it is evident that private homes are more flexible in their recruitment and deployment of staff. For example it is quite customary to appoint people to work just a few hours per week at identified periods of need. One person known to the writer works 6 hours a week in a private residential home, a further few hours as a (private) home carer, and for the remainder of the working week helps to run a family business. Pay is also lower on average in the private sector than the public sector, where staffing levels are also in general more favourable (see Sinclair et al., 1990).

Although there has been extensive research into residential care in general - invariably uncovering its inadequacies - it is worth asking why there has been so little specific interest in the paid carers. For example in a recent review of research on welfare provision for elderly people there is a chapter on informal carers, but none on paid carers in either domiciliary or residential services (Sinclair et al., 1990). Also, only one small chapter is devoted to 'Staffing of Residential Homes' in a collection of papers which brought together the main research studies commissioned by the Department of Health in the 1980s (Judge and Sinclair, 1986). This concentrates on structural issues such as staffing levels rather than on staff roles and tasks relating to the care process.

'Staffing' is discussed in 2-3 pages only in the 'The Research Reviewed' commissioned by the Wagner Committee. It is stated, 'Most research reports on old persons homes contain references to the importance of staff—These statements, however, are generally given as asides in the research reports, rather than as a result of the main research findings' (Sinclair, 1988a, p.270). The main Wagner Report, *A Positive Choice*, (Wagner, 1988), at least drew attention to the key roles played by staff at all levels by devoting two chapters (8 and 9) to staffing issues and their development and training needs respectively.

What can be stated with some degree of certainty is that the vast majority of paid carers are women and that they are on the whole low paid, often receiving (particularly in the private and voluntary sectors) far less than any envisaged minimum wage. We know too that relatively few will have been formally qualified to do the job for which they are employed, as until recently there have neither been recognised qualifications, nor the training opportunities to acquire such recognition. Nor is there any structure for career development; only a small minority are likely to rise through the ranks to become managers, for example of home care services or officers in charge of a day centre or residential home.

Some, but one suspects not in large numbers, enter care work by way of Youth Training and adult Employment Training schemes. There are also some 'special' schemes to enable people with learning disabilities to find occupation and employment in care settings. The attractions of caring, such as they are, are likely to fluctuate with the wider employment situation. We know that there is a great deal of part time working and that many paid carers are likely to live in the vicinity of their work - apart from anything else the costs of travelling would make such employment uneconomical for a great many people.

Staffing profiles thus tend to reflect the demography of an area and its local culture. For example, residential homes in areas with relatively large black populations will generally have a number of black staff. The homes themselves however are likely to reflect a predominately white culture. (For various reasons there would appear to be relatively few black people accommodated in residential homes even in areas with large ethnic communities.) It follows that issues relating to equal opportunities and racism will feature strongly in the experience of black staff and for that matter black service users, which need to be addressed on a number of levels (see, for example, Patel, 1990).

The stereotypical paid carer is a middle aged married working class woman, who transfers her experience and skills of looking after her own family, including any aged relatives to other older people, but on a paid basis. Job satisfaction comes from 'tucking people up in bed and giving them a kiss'. A survey conducted by the Social Care Association (Education), indeed, found that the largest group of residential care assistants were aged between 41 - 50 years (Social Care Association/Help the Aged, 1992).

However, attend a briefing session for home carers or step inside any residential home and it is possible to identify carers of all ages, social class and cultural backgrounds, personalities and academic abilities and qualifications. The broad age range is also supported by the Social Care Association (Education) survey, where over 30% of the sample were aged under 30 years. This also suggests that it would be unwise to generalise about care assistants' lack of abilities to perform professionally or their lack of aspirations to have greater responsibilities:

> It is our view that a significant proportion of care assistants have the potential and the commitment to form future generations of senior staff within residential care for older people. Indeed our findings suggest that a significant proportion of care assistants have ambitions for the relevant training to secure senior positions. Such potential needs to be harnessed and nurtured (Social Care Association (Education/Help the Aged, 1992, p.14).

There are still very few men employed as home carers; rather more, but not many work as care staff in residential homes and day services. But despite equal opportunities policies the further up the organisational ladder relatively more men appear in managerial positions or are home owners or managers.

ROLES AND TASKS

Home care

Traditionally, social caring for older people in their own homes has been essentially practical; providing help over tasks of daily living such as tidying up, cleaning, shopping, and preparing meals, which, usually because of physical incapacity, the person and/or partner may be unable to carry out for themselves, or can do so only with difficulty and strain. Sinclair and Williams (1990, pp.165-166) also point out that home helps are very much more likely to be provided to people living on their own; the very old, disabled and housebound; the socially disadvantaged; and to older men as against older women - when other factors are taken into account.

Personal care, i.e. help with lifting and general mobility, dressing, washing and going to the toilet, with problems such as incontinence and semi - nursing tasks, has been a relatively recent and further development of the original domestic role. The changes in role have however been formally recognised and a nationally negotiated job description includes social duties along with physical and domestic tasks.

Sinclair and Williams (1990, p.163) suggest that the key dilemma facing the organisation and management of the home care services is whether 'the service should provide large numbers of elderly people with basic cleaning and shopping on a weekly or twice weekly basis?', or 'provide fewer but more dependent people with a much more intensive and frequent service and one that includes personal care such as washing?' If the role is to include more personal care then this too has repercussions on the roles of community nurses, who would traditionally carry out such tasks in situations where they have been involved by GPs and hospital consultants.

Within community care plans, much closer integration of health and social care will be demanded and more emphasis on teamworking will be needed. The concept of community care also implies that the home care service will in general have a more sharply defined preventative function; with levels of support changing and intensifying, where necessary, in order to prevent or delay admission to more costly and less favoured residential care. This too will tend to 'upgrade' the carer's role by, for example, requiring them to be more involved in assessments and care planning processes. As Sinclair and Williams (1990, p.164) suggest, 'clients who are washed by home helps may lose contact with the medical services, so that it then becomes more important that home helps should be able to spot medical problems and refer appropriately'

With the changes in the characteristics and needs of the older population personal care has arguably become the primary caring function in home care as well as in residential and day care service settings. Indeed with the increasing resource problems facing local authorities eligibility criteria for services would seem to be tightening, virtually precluding domestic help needs on their own. Older people and their immediate carers are thus being redirected to private agencies for these services. This trend is possibly being reinforced by the charging policies of local authorities, which have the effect of making potential services users think twice about the offer of any service, even after eligibility has been established.

Residential care

In the majority of residential settings personal care, though invariably linked to associated domestic tasks, has for a long time, and continues to be regarded as the most important care function. This is seen to be the result of increasing dependency through physical and mental infirmity of residential service users. Social and emotional care have tended to be lower down the list of priorities, but are slowly being accepted as integral to the care task.

Research has suggested that the needs of older people in residential care are not, in general, that different in terms of physical dependency etc. from those who remain in their own homes and many residents are in fact quite capable of living independently with adequate and appropriate supports (See NISW Practice and Development Exchange, 1988). The inference is that admission to a residential home tends to exacerbate dependency and that care staff implicitly or explicitly encourage it through their practice and the overall regime of the home. Indeed there is some research evidence to suggest that much more is done to and for residents in homes with relatively higher staffing levels than in less well staffed homes, where residents have to do more for themselves (Power et al.,1983). This is perhaps as one would expect, and should not be taken as an argument for staff cuts! The main issue is to what ends are the 'additional' resources used.

At one level care staff certainly need to be more supportive and encouraging of residents needs and wishes for being more independent, and to have greater control over their lives; at another, the home itself should be constantly reviewing whether the individual wishes or needs to remain in its care. It follows that care staff would then need to be fully involved in the ensuing assessment, care planning and review processes and procedures, which of course adds to their range of tasks and responsibilities and for which training is required.

A further implication is for the actual functions of residential homes, which, logically, will be less the provision of permanent care, providing more flexible and individualised services that are rehabilitative in purpose and orientation. Indeed this is the direction taken by some local authority homes - exemplified by the concept of the 'resource centre'. With such changes of functions corresponding changes are needed to carers' roles, which clearly require a more 'professional' attitude and approach and development of new skills, for example, as 'key workers'. It has been suggested from one research study that to enable the formal carers to find the time to work more fully and intensively on the social and emotional care more use could be made of volunteers and informal carers to carry out the more routine tasks (Power et al., 1983). This may appear impractical, but some interesting and challenging possibilities are presented by this idea.

Taking the situation overall the position of paid carers in relation to their roles, tasks, and levels of responsibilities is a confusing one. Some continue to be employed in effectively domestic roles in home and residential settings. In some particularly smaller residential homes there is little formal or real distinction between domestic and caring roles; in others there are clear job demarcation lines. It is also interesting to note that the term 'housekeeper' is still used in some private and voluntary homes to denote the person in charge not only of domestic arrangements, but also residents' care. They are perhaps equivalent to 'Senior Care Staff' in local authorities and agencies that follow national conditions of employment and pay structures.

In residential nursing homes care assistants are employed. The assistants' work is equivalent to that of nursing auxiliaries in hospital settings and who work under the supervision of qualified nurses. In the home care services, people, who may well have been employed as home helps as traditionally defined, may now be expected to perform detailed and intimate personal care tasks as members of a community care team, possibly working closely with community nurses. This is likely to be the pattern of the foreseeable future as 'community care' is implemented.

Residential carers also are having their roles redefined and are taking on not just new tasks, but the level of complexity of their work is also changing. However, we are still a long way from achieving a unified workforce of community carers, which would include staff in residential and day services settings, envisaged by the Griffiths (1988) and Audit Commission Reports (1985; 1986).

SUPERVISION AND MANAGEMENT ROLES.

We have already stated that there is no consistent career progression for social carers working with older people. The home care service has traditionally been a very flat hierarchy with domiciliary care managers each managing and supervising large numbers of direct care workers and carrying major responsibilities for co-ordinating services with social workers and other professionals. New patterns of organisation are, however, taking shape in response to care in the community policies.

Residential and day settings tend to have more differentiated staffing structures so that there are some opportunities to progress from care assistant to senior care and officer levels. However there are major differences between public and private sectors. The private sector is partly made up of numerous small 'family businesses', where members of the owning family are likely to assume major responsibility for the running of the home. Where ownership and management are separate then managers and senior care staff will be employed, but there is no consistent organisational model followed, except possibly in the larger 'corporate' organisations, which own and manage a number of homes and which may have their own recruitment, employment and training policies.

STAFF DEVELOPMENT AND TRAINING.

Until the advent of Vocational Qualifications, which are discussed below, there has been little by way of a common training infrastructure that would assist both employers and employees to determine how to assess and meet needs. One of the main hurdles to overcome has been the lack of recognition of the need for any training. This 'training blindness' goes back a long way.

For example in their history of residential services for older people since the 1948 National Assistance Act, Means and Smith (1985) provide a fascinating account of how thinking at very high levels of policy formulation effectively prevented an acceptance of the need for training and any investment of resources in it. They refer to various reports, including one in 1952 from the Association of Municipal Corporations, which, referring to the training needs of heads of homes for older people (care assistants were not even considered), stated:

> ...it would not seem at the present time there is any need for a lengthy course (6 months had been proposed) and it is suggested that the period of training should be of not more than of two weeks duration... (Means and Smith, 1985, p.208).

The proposed contents of such training included:

- general housekeeping, 'including the purchase and storage of food in bulk; some knowledge of bulk cooking, but bearing in mind the special requirements of old people;
- special needs of old people;
- minor ailments of old people.

And that was about it! In fact it is only comparatively recently that training has been provided for other than officers - in - charge of homes or home help managers and organisers.

Compare this with a more recent analysis carried out as part of an Educational Resources project, which identified a much more comprehensive range of training needs for direct care staff. This suggested that training should begin with a planned induction programme, which should be available to everyone, not only at the beginning of a person's employment, but with any change of role, promotion or whenever the nature of the work also changes. Training should continue so that carers can gain knowledge and understanding of the people whom they are trying to help, particularly any disabilities, for example dementia, that may afflict older people. It should include some understanding of the principles of care, of the effects of life changes, for example through bereavement and loss; a good grasp of policies and procedures, and an introduction to the many different ways and means, techniques and skills of helping older people, for example through care planning, keyworking, 'reality orientation' etc. Attention should be paid to the needs of people from various ethnic groups and cultures, religions etc. Not least, training should help carers to work as effective team members (Douglas and Payne, 1988).

It is true that we have come some way to getting acknowledgement that social care with any service user group requires knowledge and skills that need to be acquired and reinforced through training and professional supervision. This recognition of the need for staff development and training has been slower in relation to services for older people. Professional supervision is still an undeveloped concept and practice, particularly one suspects in the more task orientated private sector (see Atherton, 1986).

The introduction of the Training Support Grant by the Department of Health, which initially targeted training resources on services for older people, has given a strong and much needed impetus to Local Authorities to initiate, develop and consolidate their training provision. However by and large these resources have not reached the private and voluntary sectors.

It is also true that there have been a number of courses in care provided by local colleges and other agencies, some of which have led to a recognised qualification for example, by City and Guilds, Central Council for Education and Training in Social Work, and BTech as the main awarding bodies. For managers there have also been a variety of possible training routes for example, Certificate in Social Services (CSS), Certificate of Qualification in Social Work (CQSW) and Business Management Certificates and Diplomas. But the fact has remained that there has been little or no determination as to what should be the relevant qualification for care work.

Some indeed might still argue that training and qualifications are unimportant. What counts are personal qualities and attitudes, and life experience. Thus the few surveys there have been on the numbers and percentages of staff with qualifications have invariably yielded tentative results, because of the difficulties of defining what is meant by being qualified at different levels and in identifying courses of training that lead to a 'relevant' qualification. In work with older people, for example, nursing is generally considered to be relevant experience and the possession of one or other nursing qualifications a decided advantage. This applies particularly to intensive home care and nursing homes. The possession of a nursing or social work qualification also favours people who apply for management posts, even though the corresponding training courses contain little management content.

Nursing and social care, although having much in common, are by no means identical occupations; qualifications in one do not automatically transfer to the other context. For example, Nursing Home care tends to be a combination of social and nursing care and requires additional perspectives to those associated with hospital treatment. These differences thus should be recognised in the determination of an appropriate model of training.

Training has in fact been given a much higher profile in recent years as a result of a series of reports, including the Griffiths Report into community care and reports by the Audit Commission. A National Institute for Social Work (NISW) *Research into Practice* Working Group convened to analyse research into residential care and draw out the implications for policy, practice and staff development, identified a range of training needs flowing logically from the research findings. The broad aim identified was for carers to be able to promote the recurring themes of the research studied i.e. to promote 'choice, privacy and security' . To do this entailed developing abilities:

- to contribute to assessments of needs (in a variety of contexts), including where relevant to multi-disciplinary assessments (see for example Neill, 1989);

- to observe and record; in particular to listen to the service user and identify their felt and expressed needs and wants;
- to manage conflicts of interest between clients, relatives and other people involved;
- to work with service users so that they can arrive at their own decisions;
- to identify needs for resources of different kinds and to take action to have such needs met;
- to resist pressures to take inappropriate action;
- to manage 'dependency' in its various aspects;
- to work with people suffering from various degrees of confusion and dementing illness;
- to work as a member of a team;
- to handle the more 'technical' aspects of caring e.g. medication, lifting and moving.

This was not a comprehensive list of training needs, just those that were implied by the various research findings. (NISW Practice and Development Exchange, 1988). In the next phase of work attempts were made to identify examples of 'good practice' that exemplified the research findings, i.e. to extend the range and choice of services; to develop better assessments of needs; to improve residential life etc. Change strategies that assisted the implementation of 'good practice' were also explored (see Payne, 1989a).

The Wagner Report, *A Positive Choice*, based on an independent review of residential care, recommended that every home should be required to submit and implement a training plan that included induction, some basic or foundation training, team and management training (Wagner, 1988). The Department of Health subsequently commissioned a development programme, the Caring in Homes Initiative, to demonstrate how key recommendations of the Wagner Report could be implemented. Training for Care Staff was one of the four Programmes comprising the Initiative.

As a result of this Programme training materials and practical guidance to home owners and managers have been produced from the various action research projects (see for example Mabon, 1991; Daley et al., 1992). Materials produced by other Initiative Programmes also have training aspects and implications (see for example Elkan and Kelly, 1991; Freeman and Kelly, 1992; Centre for Environmental and Studies in Ageing, 1992; Policy Studies Institute, 1992). As part of the setting up work, care staff from a number of homes were interviewed about their experiences and attitudes to training. The findings were broadly similar wherever the interviews and discussions took place, which confirm the comparative neglect of training for work with older people. Very little discussion about training needs and opportunities had ever taken place; what had been offered and attended took the form of short 'one off' courses that were soon forgotten. Training was equated with 'going to school' that occurred away from the workplace and did not necessarily relate to the job or its contents. There were few opportunities for people to reflect on and evaluate their practice and 'supervision' was by and large an alien concept (see Payne, C., 1991a; 1991b; 1992).

THE CONTRIBUTIONS OF CARERS IN CHANGING AND DEVELOPING SERVICES

Research has helped to evolve the principles that underpin service provision and delivery, and to inform influential reports such as Wagner and Griffiths and practical guidelines like *Homes Are For Living In* (DoH/SSI, 1989). In brief these principles seek to achieve the following:

- To extend the exercise of choice; eradicating the 'block treatment' and impersonal practices uncovered by much research from the seminal studies of Townsend (1962) and Goffman (1968).
- To make services more user sensitive by making them more flexible and adaptive to expressed needs and expectations This makes use of consumer research that emphasises the importance to residents of practical, everyday activities such as being able to control their immediate environment by opening and closing windows and regulating the heating in their rooms. These studies have also emphasised how much people living in both their own and residential homes value their privacy and prefer (when on their own) to have a single room (see NISW Practice and Development Exchange, 1988).
- To ensure that people in residential care are treated with dignity and respect and accorded the same 'citizens' rights as if they were living independently. People, who for reasons of mental or physical illness, are unable to exercise their rights e.g. when suffering from dementia, may require the services of an advocate or a similar arrangement.
- To ensure that they are given adequate protection from abuse and opportunities to complain about inadequate

service; there are now legal requirements to have written complaints procedures covering all services.
- To involve users more in decisions about services and to have greater control over what is provided for them.

How such principles are actually applied in practice is very much down to the front line carers and their supervisors and line managers. As work carried out for NISW as part of the 'Research into Practice' project (discussed above) and the Training for Care Staff Programme has demonstrated, change from traditional to more enlightened or progressive practice is far from easy. It is important not to underestimate what is actually required in terms of preparations, consultation, action planning and implementation. Even apparently simple changes like increasing choice of food and flexibility of mealtimes may have far reaching organisational consequences. Also good intentions may not be fulfilled in practice, as Potter and Wiseman discovered in one action research project; for example an individual's request to have salmon sandwiches for tea ended up in everyone having them! (Potter and Wiseman, 1989).

It is not surprising that some find it preferable to develop 'good practice' from scratch with new staff without other institutional experience (see, for example, Greenwell, 1989). This may be alright for new establishments, but is difficult for existing ones, where staff as a whole or indeed pockets of staff hold entrenched attitudes, which may run counter to current expectations. Here resistance to change may have to be overcome in part as a result of staff fearing that their previous and current efforts have been devalued and undermined.

Many of the Training for Care Staff projects adopted an active learning model that encouraged care staff to critically examine and evaluate how well and in what ways their current practice matched the current standards of 'Good Practice'. This made direct use of research based products such as *Homes are For Living In* (DoH/SSI, 1989) and a Self Evaluation Chart, which first appeared in *Care Weekly* (Payne, 1989b). From initial evaluations of current practice action plans were drawn up to change and improve the practice of the home in question, with some success. The processes of self evaluation, action planning and implementation are also explained more fully in a manual published jointly by the National Extension College and National Institute for Social Work (Hillyard-Parker et el., 1993).

VOCATIONAL QUALIFICATIONS .

Although taking considerable time to become established Vocational Qualifications are a considerable advance on the old 'ad hoc' arrangements. In the longer term they should contribute to a much more coherent structure of qualifications and training. The development of the VQ system has also produced other benefits. From work commissioned by the Care Sector Consortium, which is the 'Lead Industrial Body' for the social caring occupations, and the corresponding body for the National Health Service, there is now a detailed analysis of care functions and tasks as exercised in the majority of health and social care settings. This analysis has been used to underpin the Standards that people who seek to obtain NVQs must meet in their work performance.

Although the process of 'functional analysis' used to determine the standards are subject to criticism as being too 'mechanistic' to capture the nuances of skilled care (Kelly et al., 1990), the fact that they now exist represents a substantial advance on anything that has gone before. Nevertheless the production of the Standards has been tortuous. First there were separate standards for Residential and Day Care (Social Care), and Health Care respectively, which were used as interim measures for assessing competence. Then in part because of the amount of overlap between the two sets of standards a further project resulted in their integration into a single set that is now used as the common basis for VQ assessments across health and social care.

Eventually, there should be common qualifications potentially available for all carers working in community, day and residential services settings. This should allow much greater flexibility and transferability across traditional service boundaries. For example someone with VQs obtained as a nursing auxiliary should have demonstrated that they possess the basic attitudes and skills for applying to work in say a Nursing Home or Home Care situation, by virtue of the fact that they will have been assessed against certain common, 'core', value-based Standards in their previous situation. They will also have gained an 'Endorsement' that proved their competence to carry out tasks that were more situation and role specific. They could then apply to obtain further 'Endorsements', which proves their competence in their new setting and role. This theoretical flexibility and 'ladder building' potential is one of the attractions of the NVQ system.

Whether it will actually work thus will require ongoing monitoring and evaluation.

Crucial to its success as a national system will be the willingness of employers in all sectors to invest personal and financial resources in the setting up and maintenance of the quite complicated procedures entailed. To date implementation is decidedly patchy, but improving gradually.

For carers seeking qualifications the new system should be attractive. National Vocational qualifications are not strictly speaking training qualifications, but are awarded on the basis of demonstrating one's competence against defined standards. To demonstrate competence it is important to be able to display understanding and to use knowledge required of the work, but unlike a traditional college course there are no academic requirements to write essays or to pass assignments. This approach is clearly helpful to the more practical minded person, who for one reason or another might find the 'examination' approach difficult to cope with.

If the key to the NVQ assessment process is in being observably competent, the question is then how do carers learn to become competent, when for example they are assessed as 'not yet competent'? (One never actually 'fails' in NVQ assessment.) The assumption is that people can learn to become competent in all sorts of ways. So each individual will devise their own 'learning package' - with help from their assessor or a 'mentor'- that targets the specific knowledge, attitudes and skills deemed necessary to achieve competence. For some this certainly might entail attendance on a training course, or working through the contents of distance or open learning package (e.g. Open College or Open University). For others it might mean having 'tutorials' on set topics or intensive supervision and feedback on specific aspects of their practice. The main feature here is flexibility.

THE CARERS CONTRIBUTION TO THE 'COMPETENT WORKPLACE'.

As has been pointed out in an earlier study of the emerging NVQ system, 'competence' as a contribution to improving quality of service is not only about an individual person's practice and performance, but about the whole work setting and context in which individuals have to work (Kelly et al., 1990.) The notion of Standards therefore must be applied to the total service system and its management, which, arguably, must be in place as a precondition for valid assessments of individual practice and performance to be made.

This then places any system of individual qualifications and assessment into a wider context of what is becoming popularly known as 'quality assurance'. Indeed it would be difficult for any employer to consider investing in NVQ without demonstrating a commitment to overall quality, because the NVQ requirements actually demand this.

Current concepts of 'quality' of care and quality assurance processes are heavily influenced by 'provider - purchaser' relationships. The elderly person is seen as a 'consumer', who is able to exercise freely their purchasing power within the limits of their available resources and the situation in which they are placed, for example own home, residential home etc. The carers therefore should be aiming to provide a service according to the consumers' wants and one that results in 'consumer satisfaction'. The aims of the service provision are therefore to meet needs and to increase satisfaction. At a strategic level the implied aim is also to extend choice of service provision, through free market mechanisms so that different service providers may well be competing with one another in a so-called 'mixed economy' of welfare.

Following this model, 'market research' would be aimed at finding out what the 'customer' might want and expect from the service providers. For their part the providers then design their services to meet need, and expect their employees to deliver those services according to their specifications. Supervision and monitoring systems are used to determine whether they in fact do this, and the institution of complaints procedures acts as a further means of ensuring consumers have redress to faulty service.

Recently there has been a lot of interest expressed in adopting British Standards 5750 for the care sector and at the time of writing at least one home has been awarded the BS seal of approval. BS 5750 requires the institution and implementation of quality assurance systems in at least 18 aspects of practice, which individually and collectively are seen to contribute to the achievement of a 'quality assured' service. One of the criticisms of BS5750 is that it is purely a management driven process, and implementation work to date indicates that it will have value only if there is full commitment and participation of carers and service users.

A more reflective and participative model of quality assurance is provided by the Caring in Homes Initiative's Inside Quality Assurance Programme (Centre for Environmental and Social Studies in Ageing, 1992).

It is doubtful, even when community care arrangements are fully in place that the Sainsbury or Marks and Spencer 'consumerist' model can be applied wholesale to the social care of older people. There is also a danger that too rigid an application of certain aspects will be counter productive. For example the role distance, which is characteristic of shop assistant - customer relationships, if applied too strictly to carer - client or resident relationships may lead to care being experienced as clinical and impersonal. Or quality might be interpreted and measured in terms of the external features of the services, not about the more difficult to assess aspects, for example whether social and emotional needs are being addressed.

More evaluation is needed of these 'modern' service and care models. Also the implications for the day to day work of the front line carers working to these models need further working through. It is true that 'consumer' research studies have indicated that service users seek some very practical forms of help. As has already been discussed above residential life could be improved for example, by more attention being paid to, for example having a room of one's own, having opportunities to be private, being able to choose one's companions and to be able to control the immediate environment, having greater choice of food and flexibility of mealtimes.

However, research also suggests that many people in residential homes suffer considerably from loneliness and depression, as well as a range of physical and mental infirmities (Evans et al., 1981). They also frequently lack social and emotional stimulation following long periods of inactivity and boredom (Godlove et al., 1982). It is not stretching the evidence too far therefore to suggest that they need time, space and opportunities to express and have accepted these feelings about themselves and their predicament. But if the front line carers are preoccupied with the physical tasks and concentrate on the 'externals' only, like 'have you enjoyed your meal?', which is characteristic of the hotel or 'consumer' model, then these inner feelings are never going to be expressed. 'Modern' residential care will thus become only an updated version of more traditional forms of 'institutional care', physically superior, but as emotionally bleak as before.

SUMMARY

In this chapter we have examined the contributions and needs of paid carers, identifying what and how research can inform and assist the development of their practice and training. We made the point that as a focus for research, taking account the field as a whole, paid carers are a neglected species. Considerably more research is needed simply to map out more definitively the characteristics and dynamics of this large and rather unsung workforce. We then examined the range of roles and tasks expected and carried out by those on the front line of service delivery, commenting on the variations between services and settings. There is clearly a long way to go before the idea of an integrated workforce of community cares becomes a reality.

Training is self evidently a key to this development - again we need to set relatively long time horizons before expecting any substantial increase in the numbers of carers who will possess relevant qualifications. Here we are looking to vocational qualifications eventually to 'come up with the goods'.

In the later sections of the chapter we have looked at the implications of relevant research for care practice and what is needed to translate the findings into practice. This raises the issue of the whole process and methodology required for genuine and effective change and development to occur. We have referred to some action research projects, which have illuminated some of the change processes and the difficulties entailed. Further enquiry into the actual processes of changing practice towards the desired standards would certainly be fruitful.

Bibliography

Ablon, J. (1971) 'Bereavement in a Samoan community', *British Journal of Medical Psychology,* 44, pp.329-337.

Abrams, M. (1978) *Beyond Three-Score and Ten: A First Report on a Survey of the Elderly.* Mitcham, Surrey: Age Concern.

Abrams, M. (1989) 'Third age lives in the next generation: changing attitudes and expectations' in Warnes, A.M. (ed.) *Human Ageing and Later Life: Multidisciplinary Perspectives.* London: Edward Arnold.

Abrams, P. (1977) ' Community care : some research problems and priorities', *Policy and Politics,* 6(20).

Abrams, P. (1978) *Neighbourhood Care and Social Policy.* Berkhamsted: Volunteer Centre.

Adams, R. (1990) *Self-Help, Social Work and Empowerment.* London: Macmillan.

Allen, I., Hogg, D. and Peace, S. (1992) *Elderly People: Choice, Participation and Satisfaction.* London: Policy Studies Institute.

Allen, I. with Levin E., Sidell, M. and Vetter, N. (1983) 'The elderly and their informal carers' in DHSS *Research Contributions to the Development of Policy and Practice.* London: HMSO.

Antonucci, T. and Jackson, J. (1989) 'Successful ageing and life course reciprocity' in Warnes, A.M. (ed.) *Human Ageing and Later Life: Multidisciplinary Perspectives.* London: Edward Arnold.

Arber, S. and Gilbert, G.N. (1989) 'Transitions in caring: gender, life course and the care of the elderly' in Bytheway, B., Keil, T., Allatt, P. and Bryman, A. (eds.) *Becoming and Being Old: Sociological Approaches to Later Life.* London: Sage.

Archer, J.L. (1982) 'Discovering a philosophy for working with the elderly mentally infirm', *Social Work Service* , Summer, pp.43-49.

Argyle, M. and Henderson, M. (1985) *The Anatomy of Relationships.* Harmondsworth: Penguin.

Arie, T. (1991) *Women as Carers.* Paper presented at Social Gerontology Conference, Keele University.

Arling, G. (1976) 'The elderly widow and her family, neighbours and friends', Journal of Marriage and the Family, 38, pp.757-768.

Atherton, J. (1986) *Professional Supervision in Group Care. A Contract Based Approach*. London: Tavistock Publications.

Audit Commission (1985) *Managing Social Services for the Elderly More Effectively*. London: HMSO.

Audit Commission (1986) *Making a Reality of Community Care*. London: HMSO.

Baker, D.E. (1978) *Attitudes of Nurses to the Care of the Elderly*. PhD thesis, University of Manchester.

Baldwin, S.M. and Parker, G.M. (1991) 'Support for informal carers - the role of social security' in Dalley, G. (ed.) *Disability and Social Policy*. London: Policy Studies Institute.

Baltes, P.B. and Baltes, M.M. (1991) 'Psychological perspectives on successful aging: the model of selective optimization with compensation', in Baltes, P.B. and Baltes, M.M. (eds.) *Successful Aging: Perspectives from the Behavioral Sciences*. Cambridge: Cambridge University Press, pp.1-34.

Baltes, P.B., Smith, J. and Staudinger, U. (1992) 'Wisdom and successful aging', *Nebraska Symposium on Motivation*, 39, pp.123-167.

Bayley, M. (1973) *Mental Handicap and Community Care*. London: Routledge Kegan Paul.

Bhalla, A. and Blakemore, K. (1981) *Elders of the Ethnic Minority Groups*. Birmingham: AFFOR.

Blaikie, A. and Macnicol, J. (1989) 'Ageing and social policy: a twentieth century dilemma' in Warnes, A.M. (ed.) *Human Ageing and Later Life: Multidisciplinary Perspectives*. London: Edward Arnold.

Blakemore, K. (1989) 'Does age matter? the case of old age in minority ethnic groups' in Bytheway, B., Keil, T., Allatt, P. and Bryman, A. (eds.) *Becoming and Being Old: Sociological Approaches to Later Life*. London: Sage.

Blaxter, M. (1990) *Health and Lifestyles*. London: Routledge.

Bond, J. (1992) 'The future of long-term care' in Young, R. and Higginson, I.J. (eds.) *Long-Term Care for Elderly People: Purchasing, Providing and Quality*. London: HMSO.

Bond, J., Briggs, R. and Coleman, P. (1993) 'The study of ageing' in Bond, J., Coleman, P. and Peace, S. (eds.) *Ageing in Society. An Introduction to Social Gerontology*. Second Edition. London: Sage.

Bond, J. and Carstairs, V. (1982) *Services for the Elderly: A Survey of the Characteristics and Needs of a Population of 5,000 Old People*. Scottish Health Service Studies No.42. Edinburgh: Scottish Home and Health Department.

Bond, S. and Bond, J. (1990) 'Outcomes of care within a multiple-case study in the evaluation of the experimental National Health Service nursing homes', *Age and Ageing*, 19, pp.11-18.

Booth, T. (1985) *Home Truths. Old People's Homes and the Outcome of Care*. Aldershot: Gower.

Bowers, M., Jackson, E., Knight, J. and Le Shan, L. (1975) *Counselling the Dying*. New York: Aronson.

Bowlby, J. (1979) *The Making and Breaking of Affectional Bonds*. London: Tavistock.

Bowlby, J. (1985) *Loss, Sadness and Depression. Attachment and Loss*. Volume 3. Harmondsworth: Penguin.

Bowling, A. (1984) 'Caring for the elderly widowed - the burden on their supporters', *British Journal of Social Work*, 18,(5), pp.435 - 455.

Brayne, C. and Ames, D. (1988) 'The epidemiology of mental disorder in old age' in Gearing, B., Johnson, M.L. and Heller, T. (eds.) *Mental Health Problems in Old Age*. Chichester: Wiley, pp.26.

Brown, A. and Clough, R. (eds.) (1989) *Groups and Groupings*. London: Routledge.

Butler, A., Oldman, C. and Greve, J. (1983) *Sheltered Housing for the Elderly. Policy, Practise and the Consumer*. London: George Allen and Unwin.

Butler, A. with Tinker, A. (1983) 'Integration or segregation: housing in later life' in *DHSS Research Contributions to the Development of Policy and Practice*. London: HMSO.

Butler, R.N. (1963) 'The life review: an interpretation of reminiscence in the aged', *Psychiatry*, 26, pp.65-76.

Cameron, J. and Parkes, C.M. (1983) 'Terminal care: evaluation of effects on surviving family of care before and after bereavement', *Postgraduate Medical Journal*, 59, pp.73-78.

Campbell, A., Converse, P. and Rodgers, W. (eds.) (1976) *The Quality of American Life*. New York: Russell Sage Foundation.

Caplan, G. (1974) *Support Systems and Community Mental Health: Lectures on Concept Development*. New York: Behavioral Publications.

Central Statistical Office (1990) *Family Expenditure Survey 1989*. London: HMSO.

Central Statistical Office (1992) *Family Spending. A Report on the 1991 Family Expenditure Survey*. London: HMSO.

Chenoweth, B. and Spencer, B. (1986) 'Dementia: the experience of family caregivers', *The Gerontologist*, 26(3), pp.267-272.

Clark, P. and Bowling, A. (1989) Observational Study of Quality of Life in NHS Nursing Homes and a Long-Stay Ward for the Elderly, *Ageing and Society*, 9, pp.123-148.

Clifford, D. (1990) *The Social Costs and Rewards of Caring*. Avebury Studies of Care in the Community. London: Gower.

Clough, R. (1981) *Old Age Homes*. London: Allen and Unwin.

Clough, R. (1982) *Residential Work*. London: Macmillan.

Clough, R. (1986) 'Staffing of residential homes' in Judge, K. and Sinclair, I. (eds). *Residential Care for Elderly People. Research Contributions to the Development of Policy and Practice*. London: HMSO, pp.83 - 92.

Clough, R. and Parsloe, P. (eds.) (1989) *Squaring the Circle*. Bristol: University of Bristol.

Cobb, S. (1976) 'Social support as a moderator of life stress', *Psychosomatic Medicine*, 30, pp.300-314.

Cohen, S. and Wills, I.A. (1985) 'Stress, social support and the buffering hypothesis', *Psychological Bulletin*, 98, pp.310-357.

Cohler, B.J. (1982) 'Personal narrative and the life course', in Baltes, P. and Brim, O.G. Jr. (eds.) *Life-Span Development and Behavior*. Volume 4. New York: Academic Press, pp.205-241.

Cole, T.R. (1992) *The Journey of Life: A Cultural History of Aging in America*. Cambridge: Cambridge University Press.

Coleman, P.G. (1986) *Ageing and Reminiscence Processes: Social and Clinical Implications*. Chichester: Wiley.

Coleman, P.G. (1994) 'Psychological ageing' in Bond, J., Coleman, P. G and Peace, S.M. (eds.) *Ageing in Society: An Introduction to Social Gerontology*. Second Edition. London: Sage.

Coleman, P., Bond, J. and Peace, S. (1993) 'Ageing in the twentieth century' in Bond, J., Coleman, P. and Peace, S. (eds.) *Ageing in Society. An Introduction to Social Gerontology*. Second Edition. London: Sage.

Coleman, P.G. and McCulloch, A.W. (1990) 'Societal change, values and social support: exploratory studies into adjustment in late life', *Journal of Aging Studies*, 4, pp.321-332.

Colerick, E.J. and George, L.K. (1986) 'Predictors of institutionalisation among caregivers of patients with Alzheimer's disease', *Journal of the American Geriatrics Society*, 34, pp.493-498.

Cook, D. (1986) *The Influence of Participation in Reminiscence Groups on Nurses Attitudes Toward the Elderly*. MSc Thesis, Leicester University.

Coupland, N., Coupland, J. and Giles, H. (1991) *Language, Society and the Elderly: Discourse Identity and Ageing*. Oxford: Blackwell.

Cox, B.D., Blaxter, M., Buckle, A.L.J. et al. (1987) *The Health and Lifestyle Survey: Preliminary Report*. London: The Health Promotion Research Trust.

Cramond, W.A. (1970) 'Psychotherapy of the dying patient', *British Medical Journal*, 3, p.389.

Crawford, M. (1971) 'Retirement and disengagement', *Human Relations,* 24, pp.255-78.

Crawford, M. (1972) ' Retirement: a rite of passage', *Sociology,* 6, pp.477-61.

Cumming, E. and Henry, W. (1961) *Growing Old: The Process of Disengagement*. New York: Basic Books.

Dale, A., Evandrou, M. and Arber, S. (1987) 'The household structure of the elderly population in Britain', *Ageing and Society*, 7, pp.37-56.

Daley, T., Miller, T. and Wood, K. (1992) *Introduction to Care Planning* (A Training Package). London: NISW.

Dartington, T., Miller, E.J. and Gwynne, G.V. (1981) A *Life Together: The Distribution of Attitudes Around the Disabled.* London: Tavistock Publications.

Day, P.R. (1990) 'The experience of loss: the social perspective', *Changes*, 8(4), pp.304-310.

Department of the Environment, (1988) *English House Condition Survey 1986*. London: HMSO.

Department of Health (1992) *The Health of Elderly People. An Epidemiological Overview*. London: HMSO.

Department of Health/Social Services Inspectorate (1989) *Homes are for Living In.* London: HMSO.

Department of Health/Social Services Inspectorate (1990a) *Inspecting Home Care Services: A Guide to SSI Method.* London: HMSO.

Department of Health/Social Services Inspectorate (1990b) *Guidance on Standards for Residential Homes for Elderly People.* London: HMSO.

Department of Health/Social Services Inspectorate/SWSG (1991) *Care Management and Assessment: Managers' Guide.* London: HMSO.

Department of Health and Social Security (1981) *Growing Older*. Cmnd 8173. London: HMSO.

Department of Social Security, *What To Do After a Death*. Leaflet No.D49.

Department of Social Security, *Help When Someone Dies*. Leaflet No.FB29.

Dex, S. (1985) *The Sexual Division of Work, Conceptual Revolutions in the Social Sciences.* New York: St. Martin's Press.

Dittmann-Kohli, F. (1990) 'The construction of meaning in old age: possibilities and constraints', *Ageing and Society*, 10, pp.279-294.

Dittmann-Kohli, F. and Baltes, P.B. (1990) 'Toward a neofunctionalist concept of adult intellectual development: wisdom as a prototypical case of intellectual growth' in Alexander, C. and Langer, E. (eds.) *Higher Stages of Human Development*. New York: Oxford University Press, pp.54-77.

Douglas, R. and Payne, C. (1988) *Organising for Learning. Staff Development Strategies for Residential and Day Services Work. A Theoretical and Practical Guide*. London: NISW.

Eastman, M. (1984) *Old Age Abuse*. London: Age Concern.

Education Guardian (1992) 'Who cares?', 12 May.

Elkan, R. and Kelly, D. (1991) *A Window in Homes - Literature Review*. Social Care Association (Education).

Equal Opportunities Commission (1980) *The Experience of Caring for Elderly and Handicapped Dependants*. Manchester: EOC.

Erikson, E. (1950) *Childhood and Society*. New York: Norton.

Erikson, E. (1965) *Childhood and Society*. New York: Norton.

Erikson, E.H. (1978) 'Reflections on Dr Borg's life cycle' in Erikson, E.H. (ed.) *Adulthood*. New York: Norton.

Erikson, E.H., Erikson, J.M. and Kivnick, H.Q. (1986) *Vital Involvement in Old Age: The Experience of Old Age in Our Time*. New York: Norton.

Evandrou, M. and Victor, C.R. (1989) 'Differentiation in later life: social class and housing tenure cleavages' in Bytheway, B., Keil, T., Allatt, P. and Bryman, A. (eds.) *Becoming and Being Old: Sociological Approaches to Later Life*. London: Sage.

Evans, B., Hughes, B. and Wilkin, D. with Jolley, P (1981) *The Management of Mental and Physical Impairment in Non-Specialist Residential Homes for the Elderly*. University of Manchester Department of Psychiatry and Community Medicine.

Evers, H.K. (1981) 'The creation of patient careers in geriatric wards: aspects of policy and practice', *Social Science and Medicine*, 15A, pp.581-588.

Everitt, D.E., Fields, D.R., Soumerai, S.S. and Avorn, J. (1991) 'Resident behaviour and staff distress in the nursing home', *Journal of the American Geriatrics Society*, 39(8), pp.792-798.

Featherstone, M. and Hepworth, M. (1989) 'Ageing and old age: reflections on the postmodern life course' in Bytheway, B., Keil, T., Allatt, P. and Bryman, A. (eds.) *Becoming and Being Old: Sociological Approaches to Later Life*. London: Sage.

Featherstone, M. and Hepworth, M. (1993) 'Images of Ageing' in Bond, J., Coleman, P. and Peace, S. (eds.) *Ageing in Society. An Introduction to Social Gerontology*. Second Edition. London: Sage.

Fennell, G., Phillipson, C. and Evers, H. (1988) *The Sociology of Old Age*. Milton Keynes, Bucks: Open University Press.

Fenton, S. (1986) *Health and Welfare: Afro Caribbean and South Asian People in Central Bristol: Health and Social Services*. Unpublished Report. Department of Sociology, University of Bristol.

Field, D. and Millsap, R.E. (1991) 'Personality in advanced old age: continuity or change?', *Journal of Gerontology*, 46, pp.299-308.

Finch, J. (1984) 'Community care: developing non-sexist alternatives', *Critical Social Policy*, 9, pp.6 -18.

Fischer, D.H. (1978) *Growing Old in America*. New York: Oxford University Press.

Fletcher, P. (1991) *The Future of Sheltered Housing - Who Cares. Policy Report*. London: National Federation of Housing Associations.

Francis, D. (1984) *Will You Still Need Me, Will You Still Feed Me, When I'm 84?* Bloomington: Indiana University Press.

Freeman, K. and Kelly, D. (1992) *Widening Horizons Practice Guide*. Social Care Association (Education).

Gearing, B. and Dant, T. (1990) 'Doing biographical research' in Peace, S.M. (ed.) *Researching Social Gerontology: Concepts, Methods and Issues*. London: Sage, pp.143-159.

Gershon, S. and Hermon, S.P. (1982) 'The differential diagnosis of dementia', *Journal of the American Geriatrics Society*, Supplement, 30(11), pp.58-65.

Gilleard, C.J., Gilleard, E. and Whittick, J.E. (1984) 'Impact of psychogeriatric day hospital on the patient's family', *British Journal of Psychiatry*, 145, pp.487 - 492.

Gilligan, C. (1982) *In a Different Voice: Psychological Theory and Women's Development*. Cambridge, Mass and London: Harvard University Press.

Glaser, B.G. and Strauss, A.L. (1968) *Time for Dying*. Chicago: Aldric.

Godlove, C., Richard, L. and Rodwell, G. (1982) *Time for Action. An Observation Study of Elderly People in 4 Different Care Environments*. University of Sheffield : Joint Unit For Social Services Research.

Goffman, E. (1961) *Asylum: Essays on the Social Situation of Mental Patients and Other Inmates*. New York: Anchor/Doubleday.

Goffman, E. (1968) *Asylums, Essays of the Social Situation of Mental Patients, and Other Inmates*. Harmondsworth: Penguin.

Goldberg, E. and Hatch, S. (eds.) (1981) *A New Look at the Personal Social Services*. London; Policy Studies Institute, London.

Goldberg, E.M. and Connolly, N. (1982) *The Effectiveness of Social Care for the Elderly: An Overview of Recent and Current Evaluative Research*. London: Heinemann for the Policy Studies Institute.

Goldstein, H. (1973) *Social Work Practice: A Unitary Approach* Columbia, South Carolina: University of South Carolina Press.

Gorer, G. D. (1965) *Death, Grief and Mourning in Contemporary Britain*. London: Cresset.

Graham, H. (1991) 'The concept of caring in feminist research: the case of domestic service', *Sociology*, 25(1), pp.61-78.

Graham, H. (1983) 'Caring: a labour of love' in Finch, J. and Groves, D. (eds.) *A Labour of Love: Women, Work and Caring*. London: Routledge and Kegan Paul.

Gramlich, E. P. (1968) 'Recognition and management of grief in elderly patients', *Geriatrics*, 23, pp.87-92.

Green, H. (1988) *Informal Carers*. London: HMSO.

Greenwell, S. (1989) *Whose Home Is It Anyway? An Action Research Project Surrounding the Development of a Residential and Day Care Facility for Older People*. University of Bath School of Social Sciences.

Griffiths, R. (1988) *Community Care. Agenda for Action*. Report to the Secretary for State for Social Services by Sir Roy Griffiths. London: HMSO.

Groombridge, B. (1989) 'Education and later life' in Warnes, A.M. (ed.) *Human Ageing and Later Life: Multidisciplinary Perspectives*. London: Edward Arnold.

Gubrium, J. (1973) *The Myth of the Golden Years*. Springfield: Thomas.

Gurland, B. J. (1976) 'The comparative frequency of depression in various adult age groups', *Journal of Gerontology*, 31, pp.283-292.

Gutmann, D.L. (1987) *Reclaimed Powers: Towards a New Psychology of Men and Women in Later Life*. New York: Basic Books.

Handy, C. (1989) *The Age of Unreason*. London: Business Books.

Hanvey, C. (1989) 'Death in residence' in Philpot, T. (ed.) *Last Things*. London: Community Care.

Hazan, H. (1980) *The Limbo People: A Study of the Constitution of the Time Universe Among the Aged*. London: Routledge and Kegan Paul.

Haight, B.K. (1988) 'The therapeutic role of a structured life review process in homebound elderly subjects', *Journal of Gerontology*, 43, pp.40-44.

Heim, A. (1990) *Where Did I Put My Spectacles?* Cambridge: Allborough Press.

Henderson, A.S. (1989) 'Psychiatric epidemiology and the elderly', *International Journal of Geriatric Psychiatry*, 4, pp.249-253.

Henwood, M. and Wicks, M. (1984) *The Forgotten Army: Family Care and Elderly People*. London: Family Policy Studies Centre.

Hill, S. (1969) *A Change for the Better*. London: Hamish Hamilton.

Hillyard-Parker, H. Mabon, G. Payne, C. Phillipson, J. and Riley, M. (1993) *How to Manage Your Training. Developing a Training Plan*. National Extension College/ National Institute for Social Work.

Hinton, J. (1972) *Dying*. Harmondsworth: Penguin.

Hipkiss, A. and Bittles, A. (1989) 'Basic biological aspects of ageing' in Warnes, A.M. (ed.) *Human Ageing and Later Life: Multidisciplinary Perspectives*. London: Edward Arnold.

Hipkiss, A. (1989) 'The production and removal of abnormal proteins: a key question in the biology of ageing' in Warnes, A.M. (ed.) *Human*

Ageing and Later Life: Multidisciplinary Perspectives. London: Edward Arnold.

Hockey, J. and James, A. (1990) *Metaphors of Marginality: Ageing, Infantilisation and Personhood.* Paper presented at British Society of Gerontology Annual Conference,Durham 21-23 September 1990.

Hollis, F. and Woods, M.E. (1981) *Casework: A Psychosocial Therapy.* New York: Random House.

Hope, R. and Fairburn, C.G. (1990) 'The nature of wandering: a community based study'. *International Journal of Geriatric Psychiatry*, 5, pp.239-245.

House of Commons, (1990) *Parliamentary Debates* (Hansard). Sixth Series, Volume 177. London: HMSO.

Hunt, A. (1968) *Women's Employment.* London: HMSO.

Hunt, A. (1978) *The Elderly at Home.* London: HMSO.

Hussian, R.A. (1990) 'Stimulus control in the modification of problematic behaviour in elderly institutionalised patients', *International Journal of Behavioural Geriatrics*, 1(1), pp.33-42.

Hussian, R.A. and Brown, D.C. (1987) 'Use of two-dimensional grid patterns to limit hazardous ambulation in demented patients', *Journal of Gerontology*, 42(5), pp.558-560.

Jerrome, D. (1993) 'Intimate relationships' in Bond, J., Coleman, P. and Peace, S. (eds.) *Ageing in Society. An Introduction to Social Gerontology.* Second Edition. London: Sage.

Jones, D.A. and Vetter, N. (1984) 'A survey of those who care for the elderly at home: their problems and needs', *Social Science and Medicine*, 19(5), pp.511-514.

Jones, K. and Fowles, A. (1984) *Ideas on Institutions.* Routledge and Kegan Paul.

Jorm, A.F. (1990) *The Epidemiology of Alzheimer's Disease and Related Disorders.* London: Chapman and Hall.

Judge, K. and Sinclair, I (eds.) (1986) *Residential Care for Elderly People. Research Contributions to the Development of Policy and Prarctice.* London: HMSO.

Jung, C.G. (1972) 'The transcendent function' in Read, H., Fordham, M., Adler, G. and McGuire, W. (eds.) *The Structure and Dynamics of the Psyche.* Second Edition, Volume 8 of the Collected Works of C.G. Jung. London: Routledge and Kegan Paul.

Kalish, R. A. (1978) 'A little myth is a dangerous thing: research in the service of the dying' in Garfield, C.A. (ed.) *Psychosocial Care of the Dying Patient.* New York: McGraw Hill.

Kalish, R.A. and Reynolds, D.K. (1977) 'The role of age in death attitudes', *Death Education*, 1, pp.205-30.

Karn, V. (1977) *Retiring to the Seaside.* London: Routledge and Kegan Paul.

Kastenbaum, R. (1969) 'Death and bereavement in later life' in Kutschen, A.H. (ed.) *Death and Bereavement*. Springfield, Illinois: Charles Thomas.

Kaufman, S.R. (1987) *The Ageless Self: Sources of Meaning in Late Life*. Madison: University of Wisconsin Press.

Kay, D.W.K., Beamish, P. and Roth, M. (1964) 'Old age mental disorders in Newcastle Upon Tyne. Part 1: a study of prevalence', *British Journal of Psychiatry*, 110, pp.146-158.

Keith, D.M. (1979) 'Life changes and perceptions of life and death among older men and women', *Journal of Gerontology*, 34, pp.870-878.

Kelly, D. ,Payne, C. and Warwick, J. (1990) *Making National Vocational Qualifications Work for Social Care*. London: NISW.

Kitwood, T. (1990) 'The dialectics of dementia: with particular reference to Alzheimer's disease', *Ageing and Society*, 10, pp.177-196.

Kivnick, H.Q. (1991) *Living with Care, Caring for Life: The Inventory of Life Strengths*. Minneapolis: School of Social Work, University of Minnesota.

Koenig, H.G. (1992) *Successful Aging, Religion and Mental Health*. New York: Haworth Press.

Kubler Ross, E. (1970) *On Death and Dying*. London: Tavistock.

Laczko, F. and Phillipson, C. (1991) *Changing Work and Retirement*. Buckingham: Open University Press.

Laing, W. and Buisson (1992) *Laing and Buisson Review of Private Health Care*. London: Laing and Buisson.

Langer, E.J. (1989) 'Minding matters: the consequences of mindlessness-mindfulness', *Advances in Experimental Social Psychology*, 22, pp.137-175.

Laslett, P.A. (1989) *A Fresh Map of Life: The Emergence of the Third Age*. London: Weidenfeld and Nicolson.

Law, C.M. and Warnes, A.M. (1982) 'The destination decision in retirement migration' in Warnes, A.M. (ed.) *Geographical Perspectives on the Elderly*. Chichester: Wiley, pp.53-81.

Law, C.M. and Warnes, A.M. (1985) 'Elderly population distribution and housing prospects in Britain', *Town Planning Review*, 56, pp.292-314.

Lendrum, S. and Syme, G. (1992) *Gift of Tears. A Practical Approach to Loss and Bereavement Counselling*. London: Tavistock-Routledge.

Levin, E., Sinclair, I. and Gorbach, P. (1983) *The Supporters of Confused Elderly People at Home*. Extract from the Main Report. London: NISW Research Unit.

Levin, E., Sinclair, I.A.C. and Gorbach, P. (1989) *Families, Services and Confusion in Old Age*. Aldershot: Gower.

Lewis, J. and Meredith, B. (1988) 'Daughters caring for mothers: the experience of caring and its implications for professional helpers', *Ageing and Society*, 8(1), pp.1 -21.

Lichtenberg, P.A. and Strzepak, D.M. (1990) 'Assessment of institutionalised dementia patients competencies to participate in intimate relationships', *The Gerontologist*, 30(1), pp.117-120.

Lieberman, M.A. and Tobin, S.S. (1983) *The Experience of Old Age: Stress, Coping and Survival*. New York: Basic Books.

Lindemann, E. (1944) 'Symptomatology and management of acute grief', *American Journal of Psychiatry*, 10, pp.141-48.

Lindemann, E. (1979) *Beyond Grief: Studies in Crisis Intervention*. New York: Aronson.

Litz, B.T., Zeiss, A.M. and Davies, H.D. (1990) 'Sexual concerns of male spouses of female Alzheimer's patients', *The Gerontologist*, 30(1), pp.13-117.

Local Government Management Board (LGMB) Employment Surveys and Research Unit (1991) *Social Services Workforce Analysis Handbook. Report Commissioned by the Social Services Inspectorate*. London: LGMB.

Lopata, H.Z. (1979) *Women as Widows: Support Systems*. New York: Elsevier.

Lynch, J.J. (1977) *The Broken Heart: The Medical Consequences of Loneliness*. New York: Basic Books.

Mabon, G. (1991) *An Induction Programme*. London: NISW.

MacFarlane, A. (1986) *Marriage and Love in England: Modes of Reproduction 1300-1840*. Oxford: Basil Blackwell.

Macintyre, S. (1977) 'Old age as a social problem' in Dingwall, R., Health, C., Reid, M. and Stacey, M. (eds.) *Health Care and Health Knowledge*. London: Croom Helm, pp.41-63.

Marris, P. (1986) *Loss and Change*. London: Routledge and Kegan Paul.

Marshall, M. (ed.) (1990) *Working with Dementia: Guidelines for Professionals*. Birmingham: Venture Press.

Martin, J., Meltzer, H. and Elliot, D. (1988) *Office of Population Censuses and Surveys Disability Surveys, Report 1: The Prevalence of Disability Among Adults*. London: HMSO.

Martin, J. and Roberts, C. (1984) *Women and Employment: A Lifetime Perspective*. London: HMSO.

Martin, J., White, A. and Meltzer, H. (1989) *Disabled Adults: Services, Transport and Employment*. London: HMSO.

McAdams, D.P. (1990) *The Person: An Introduction to Personality Psychology*. San Diego: Harcourt Brace Jovanovich.

McCrae, R.R. and Costa, P.T. (1990) *Personality in Adulthood*. New York: Guilford Press.

McNeill-Taylor, L. (1983) *Living with Loss, A Book for the Widowed.* Glasgow: Fontana.

Meddaugh, D.I. (1990) 'Reactance: understanding aggressive behaviour in long-term care', *Journal of Psychosocial Nursing and Mental Health Services*, 28(4), pp.28-33.

Miles, A. (1991) *Women, Health and Medicine.* Milton Keynes: Open University Press.

Miller, E.J. and Gwynne, G.V. (1972) *A Life Apart. A Pilot Study of Residential Institutions for the Physically Handicapped and the Young Chronic Sick.* London: Tavistock Publications.

Minois, G. (1989) *History of Old Age: From Antiquity to the Renaissance.* Cambridge: Polity Press.

Moody, H.R. (1984) 'Reminiscence and the recovery of the public world', in Kaminsky, M. (ed.) *The Uses of Reminiscence.* New York: Haworth Press.

Morrant, J.C. and Ablog, J.R. (1983) Anger in the Elderley, Postgraduate Medicine 74(6), pp,93-102

Moroney, R.M. (1976) *The Family and the State: Considerations for Social Policy.* London: Longman.

Munnichs, J.M. (1966) *Old Age and Finitude: A Contribution to Psychogerontology.* Basle: Karger.

Munnichs, J,M. (1992) 'Ageing: a kind of autobiography', *European Journal of Gerontology*, 2, pp.244-250.

Murray, H.A. (1938) *Explorations in Personality.* New York: Oxford University Press.

Naylor, G.F.K. and Harwood, E. (1975) 'Old dogs, new tricks: age and ability', *Psychology Today*, 1, pp.29-33.

Neill, J. (1989) *Assessing Elderly People For Residential Care. A Practical Guide.* London: National Institute for Social Work.

Neugarten, B.L. (ed.) (1988a) *Personality in Middle and Later Life.* New York: Atherton Press.

Neugarten, B.L. (1988b) 'Personality and psychosocial patterns of aging' in Bergener, M., Ermini, M. and Stahelin, H.B. (eds.) *Crossroads in Aging.* London: Academic Press, pp.205-218.

Neugarten, B.L., Havighurst, R.J. and Tobin, S.S. (1961) 'The measurement of life satisfaction', *Journal of Gerontology*, 16, pp.134-143.

National Institute for Social Work Practice and Development Exchange (1988) *Residential Care for Elderly People: Using Research to Improve Practice. Report of a Working Group* . London: National Institute for Social Work.

Norris, A. (1986) *Reminiscence with Elderly People.* Winslow Press.

Office of Population Censuses and Surveys (1982) *General Household Survey 1980.* London: HMSO.

Office of Population Censuses and Surveys (1988) *General Household Survey 1985*. London: HMSO.

Office of Population Censuses and Surveys (1990) *General Household Survey 1988*. London: HMSO.

Office of Population Censuses and Surveys (1991) *National Population Projections 1989-Based*. Series PP2, No. 17. London: HMSO.

Office of Population Censuses and Surveys and Registrar General Scotland (1983) *Census 1981. Persons of Pensionable Age. Great Britain*. London: HMSO.

Oswin, M. (1991) 'Don't ask us to dance (some aspects of bereavement for people who have learning difficulties' in Newnes, C. (ed.) *Death, Dying and Society*. Hove and London: Lawrence Erlbaum Associates.

Parker, G. (1990) *With Due Care and Attention: A Review of Research on Informal Care*. London: Family Policy Studies Centre.Second Edition.

Parker, R. (1981) 'Tending and social policy' in Goldberg, E.M. and Hatch, S. (eds.) *A New Look at the Personal Social Services*. London: Policy Studies Institute.

Parkes, C.M. and Weiss, R.S. (1983) *Recovery from Bereavement*. New York: Basic Books.

Parsloe, P. (1989) in Clough, R. and Parsloe, P. (eds) *Squaring the Circle*. Bristol: University of Bristol.

Patel, N. (1990) *A 'Race' Against Time? Social Service Provision to Black Elders*. The Runnymede Trust.

Payne, C. (1989a) *Better Services for Older People*. London: National Institute for Social Work.

Payne, C. (1989b) 'In our own hands. The NISW/*Care Weekly* guide to self evaluation', *Care Weekly*, 19 May, pp 13-16.

Payne, C. (1991a) 'Development - the key to effective training?', *The Journal of Training and Development*. 1(4), Feb, pp.6-17.

Payne, C. (1991b) 'Training for care staff development programme: some initial findings', *The Journal of Training and Development*, 2(2), Oct, pp 3-24.

Payne, M. (1986) *Social Care in the Community*. London: Macmillan.

Payne, M. (1991) *Modern Social Work Theory: A Critical Introduction*. London: Macmillan.

Payne, M. (1993) *Linkages: Effective Networking in Social Care*. London: Whiting and Birch/SCA.

Peace, S. (1986) 'The forgotten female: social policy and older women' in Phillipson, C. and Walker, A. (eds.) *Ageing and Social Policy - A Critical Assessment*. London: Gower.

Peters, T. and Austin, N. (1985) *A Passion for Excellence*. New York: Random House.

Peters, T. and Waterman, R. (1982) *In Search of Excellence*. New York: Harper and Row.

Phillipson, C. (1982) *Capitalism and the Construction of Old Age*. London: Macmillan.

Phillipson, C. (1987) 'The transition to retirement' in Cohen, G. (ed.) *Social Change and the Life Course*. London: Tavistock.

Phillipson, C. (1993) 'The Sociology of Retirement' in Bond, J., Coleman, P. and Peace, S. (eds.) *Ageing in Society. An Introduction to Social Gerontology*. Second Edition. London: Sage.

Philpot, T. (ed.) (1989) *Last Things*. London: Community Care.

Pilley, C. (1990) *Adult Education, Community Development and Older People: Releasing the Resource*. London: Cassell/Council of Europe.

Pincus, A. and Minahan, A. (1973) *Social Work Practice: Model and Method*. Itasca. Ill: Peacock.

Pincus, L. (1976) *Death and the Family*. London: Faber and Faber.

Pinkston, E.M. and Linsk, N.L. (1984) *Care of the Elderly: A Family Approach*. New York: Pergamon.

Policy Studies Institute (1992) *Home Truths*. Policy Studies Institute.

Potter, P. and Wiseman, V. (1989) *Improving Residential Practice: Promoting Choice in Homes for Elderly People*. London: National Institute for Social Work Practice and Development Exchange.

Power, M., Clough, R., Gibson, P. and Kelly, S. (1983) *Helping Lively Minds. Volunteer Support to Residential Homes Social Care Research*. Bristol: University of Bristol.

Pruyser, P.W. (1975) 'Aging: downward, upward or forward?' in Hiltner, S. (ed.) *Towards a Theology of Aging*. New York: Human Sciences Press, pp.102-118.

Qureshi, H. (1990) 'Formal and informal care-giving work' in Ungerson C. (ed.) *Gender and Caring*. Hemel Hempstead: Harvester Wheatsheaf.

Qureshi, H. and Walker, A. (1986) 'Caring for elderly people: the family and the state' in Phillipson, C. and Walker, A. (eds.) *Ageing and Social Policy - A Critical Assessment*. London: Gower.

Rabins, P.V., Mace, N.L. and Lucas, M.J. (1982) 'The impact of dementia on the family', *Journal of the American Medical Association*, 248, pp.333-335.

Reid, W.J. (1978) *The Task-Centered System*. New York: Columbia University Press.

Robinson, C. (1991) *Home and Away: Respite Care in the Community*. Birmingham: Venture Press.

Rochford, G. (1985) 'Bereavement' in Lishman, J. (ed.) *Developing Services for the Elderly*. London: Kogan Page.

Rodabough, T. (1980) 'Alternatives to the stages model of the dying process', *Death Education*, 4, pp.1-19.

Rodin, J. (1986) 'Aging and health: effects of the sense of control', *Science*, 233, pp.1271-1276.

Rose, S.M. and Black, B.L. (1985) *Advocacy and Empowerment: Mental Health Care in the Community*. Boston: Routledge and Kegan Paul.

Ryden, M. (1988) 'Aggressive behaviour in persons with dementia living in the community', *The Alzheimer Disease and Associated Disorders: International Journal*, 30(2), pp.206-211.

Ryff, C.D. and Heincke, S.G. (1983) 'Subjective organisation of personality in adulthood and aging', *Journal of Personality and Social Psychology*, 44, pp.807-816.

Sarason, I.G., Levine, H.M., Basham, R.B. and Sarason, B. (1983) 'Assessing social support: the social support questionnaire, *Journal of Personality and Social Psychology*, 44, pp.127-39.

Schaie, K.W. (1990) 'The optimization of cognitive functioning in old age: predictions based on cohort-sequential and longitudinal data' in Baltes, P.B. and Baltes, M.M. (eds.) *Successful Aging: Perspectives from the Behavioral Sciences*. Cambridge: Cambridge University Press, pp. 94-117.

Scrutton, S. (1989) *Counselling Older People*. London: Edward Arnold.

Secretaries of State for Health, Social Security, Wales and Scotland (1989) *Caring for People. Community Care in the Next Decade and Beyond.* CM849,White Paper. London: HMSO.

Seyd, R, Tennant, A. and Bayley, M. (1983) *The Home Help Services.* Paper 6. Dinnington Neighbourhood Services Project, Department of Sociological Studies, University of Sheffield.

Sheldon, J. (1948) *The Social Medicine of Old Age*. London: Oxford University Press.

Sinclair, I. (1988) 'Residential care for elderly people' in Sinclair, I. (ed.) *Residential Care: The Research Reviewed.* Literature surveys commissioned by the Independent Review of Residential Care. London: HMSO.

Sinclair, I. (ed.) (1988) *Residential Care: The Research Reviewed.* London: HMSO.

Sinclair, I. (1990) 'Carers: their contribution and quality of life' in Sinclair, I., Parker, R., Leat, D. and Williams ,J. (eds.) *The Kaleidoscope of Care. A Review of Research on Welfare Provision for Elderly People.* London: HMSO.

Sinclair, I. et al. (1988) *Bridging Two Worlds*. London: Avebury.

Sinclair, I., Crosbie, D., O'Connor, P., Stanforth, L. and Vickery, A. (1984) *A Study of Informal Care Services and Social Work for Elderly Clients Living Alone.* National Institute for Social Work Research Unit.

Sinclair, I., Parker, R., Leat, D. and Williams, J. (1990) *The Kaleidoscope of Care: A Review of Research on Welfare Provision for Elderly People.* London: HMSO.

Smith, C.R. (1982) *Social Work with the Dying and Bereaved.* London: MacMillan.

Social Care Association (Education)/Help the Aged (1992) *The Lost Potential. A Project Report on Care Assistants Working with Older People in Residential Settings.* SCA (Education)/ Help the Aged.

Solomon, B.B. (1976) *Black Empowerment: Social Work in Oppressed Communities.* New York: Columbia University Press.

Strehler, B.L. (1962) *Time, Cells and Aging.* New York: Academic Press.

Sudnow, D. (1967) *Passing On - The Social Organisation of Dying.* Englewood Cliffs, N.J: Practice Hall.

Swift, C. (1989) 'Health care of the elderly: the concept of progress' in Warnes, A.M. (ed.) *Human Ageing and Later Life: Multidisciplinary Perspectives.* London: Edward Arnold.

Taylor, S.E. (1979) 'Hospital patient behaviour: Reactance, helplessness or control?', *Journal of Social Issues*, 35, pp.156-184.

Thomson, D. (1983) 'Workhouse to nursing home: residential care of elderly people in England since 1840', *Ageing and Society*, 3, pp.41-69.

Tinker, A. (1984) *Staying at Home: Helping Elderly People.* London: HMSO.

Tinker, A. with Abrams, M., Muir Grey, J. and Rowlings, C. (1983) 'Improving the quality of life and promoting independence of elderly people' in *DHSS Research Contributions to the Development of Policy and Practice.* London: HMSO.

Tobin, S.S. (1991) *Personhood in Advanced Old Age: Implications for Practice.* New York: Springer.

Tobin, S. and Lieberman, M. (1976) *Last Home for the Aged.* San Francisco: Jossey-Bass.

Townsend, P. (1957) *The Family Life of Old People.* London: Routledge and Kegan.

Townsend, P. (1962) *The Last Refuge - A Survey of Residential Institutions and Homes for the Aged in England and Wales.* London: Routledge and Kegan.

Townsend, P. (1963) *The Family Life of Old People.* Harmondsworth: Penguin.

Townsend, P. (1979) *Poverty in the United Kingdom: A Survey of Household Resources and Standards of Living.* Harmondsworth: Penguin.

Townsend, P. (1981) 'The structured dependency of the elderly: a creation of social policy in the twentieth century', *Ageing and Society*, 1, pp.5-28.

Townsend, P. (1986) 'Ageism and social policy' in Phillipson, C. and Walker, A. (eds.) *Ageing and Social Policy: A Critical Assessment.* Aldershot: Gower.

Townsend, P. and Wedderburn, D. (1965) *The Aged in the Welfare State*. London: Bell and Sons.

Twining, C. (1988) *Helping Older People: A Psychological Approach.* John Wiley and Sons.

Ungerson, C. (1987) *Policy is Personal: Sex, Gender and Informal Care.* London and New York: Tavistock.

Victor, C. (1991) *Health and Health Care in Later Life.* Milton Keynes: Open University Press.

Victor, C.R. (1987) Old *Age in Modern Society: A Textbook of Social Gerontology*. London: Croom Helm.

Waerness, K. (1990) 'Informal and formal care in old age' in Ungerson, C. (ed.) *Gender and Caring.* Hemel Hempstead: Harvester Wheatsheaf.

Wagner, G. (1988) *Residential Care: A Positive Choice.* Report of the Independent Review of Residential Care. London: HMSO.

Walker, A. (1982) 'Dependency and old age', *Social Policy and Administration*, 16, pp.115-135.

Walker, A. (1993) 'Poverty and Inequality in Old Age' in Bond, J., Coleman, P. and Peace, S. (eds.) *Ageing in Society. An Introduction to Social Gerontology*. Second Edition. London: Sage.

Walker, A. and Phillipson, C. (1986) 'Introduction' in Phillipson, C, and Walker, A. (eds.) *Ageing and Social Policy. A Critical Assessment.* Aldershot: Gower, pp.1-12.

Walker, G. (1990) *With Due Care and Attention: A Review of Research on Informal Care.* Occasional Paper 2. London: Family Policy Studies Centre.

Walton, R.G. (ed.) (1986) 'Integrating formal and informal care - the utilization of social support networks', *British Journal of Social Work,* 16, Supplement.

Wass, H. and Myers, J. (1985) 'Psycho-social aspects of death among the elderly: a review of the literature' in Bloom, M. (ed.) *Life Span Development*. New York: MacMillan.

Weale, R. (1989) 'Eyes and age: views on visual health promotion' in Warnes, A.M. (ed.) *Human Ageing and Later Life: Multidisciplinary Perspectives.* London: Edward Arnold.

Wells, N. and Freer, C. (1988) *The Ageing Population: Burden or Challenge?* Basingstoke: Macmillan.

Ware, C.J.G., Fairburn, C.G. and Hope, R.A. (1990) 'A community based study of aggressive behaviour in dementia', *International Journal of Geriatric Psychiatry*, 5, pp.337-342.

Wenger, G.C. (1984) *The Supportive Network.* London: Allen and Unwin.

West, P., Illsley, R. and Kellman, H. (1984) 'Public preferences for the care of dependency groups', *Social Science and Medicine,* 18(4), pp.287 - 295.

Whittaker, J.K. and Garbarino, J. (eds.) (1983) *Social Support Networks: Informal Helping in the Human Services.* New York: Aldine.

Willcocks, D., Peace, S. and Kellaher, L. (1987) *Private Lives in Public Places: A Research-Based Critique of Residential Life in Local Authority Old People's Homes. London: Tavistock.*

Williams, J. (1990) in Sinclair, I., Parker, R., Leat, D. and Williams, J. *Kaleidoscope of Care. A Review of Research on Welfare Provisions for Elderly People.* London: HMSO.

Willmott, P. and Young, M. (1960) *Family and Class in a London Suburb.* London: Routledge and Kegan Paul.

Wolins, M. (1982) *Revitalising Residential Settings.* San Francisco: Jossey-Bass.

Woods, R.T. and Britton, P.G. (1985) Clinical Psychology with the Elderly. London: Croom Helm.

Worden, W. (1983) *Grief Counselling and Grief Therapy.* London: Tavistock.

Wright, L.K. (1991) 'The impact of Alzheimer's disease on the marital relationship', *The Gerontologist,* 31(2), pp.224-237.

Yamomoto, J., Okanogi, K., Iwasaki, T. and Toshimura, S. (1969) 'Mourning in Japan', *American Journal of Psychiatry,* 125, pp.1660-65.

Young, M. and Willmott, P. (1957) *Family and Kinship in East London.* London: Routledge and Kegan Paul.

Contributors

John Bond is Senior Lecturer in Sociology and Director of Research, Centre for Health Services Research, University of Newcastle upon Tyne.

Roger J. Clough is Chief Inspector of Social Services, Cumbria County Council. Formerly Senior Lecturer in Social Work, University of Bristol, with a special interest in residential work. His book *Old Age Homes* sets out what it is like to live and to work in a residential home for older people.

Peter G. Coleman is Professor of Social Gerontology, Departments of Geriatric Medicine and Social Work Studies, University of Southampton.

Peter R. Day is Visiting Fellow, Centre for Research in Social Policy, Department of Social Sciences, Loughborough University of Technology, formerly Lecturer in Social Work, Hull University. He has practice experience as a hospital social worker and at St Barnabas Hospice, Lincoln.

Margaret A. Fielden is Principal Clinical Psychologist, Southern Derbyshire Mental Health Trust. Formerly Head of Elderly Speciality Clinical Psychology Services, South East Staffordshire Health Authority (Premier Health NHS Trust); and Lecturer, Departments of Psychiatry and Social Gerontology, Keele University.

Chris Payne is Consultant in Social Care, National Institute for Social Work; Co-ordinator, Centre for Practical and Staff Development, University of Warwick Science Park.

Malcolm Payne is Professor and Head of Department of Applied Community Studies, The Manchester Metropolitan University.

Judith Unell is an Independent Researcher; Research Associate, Centre for Research in Social Policy, Loughborough University; and Consultant to Charities Evaluation Services.

www.ingramcontent.com/pod-product-compliance
Lightning Source LLC
LaVergne TN
LVHW101502200926
848483LV00001B/201
* 9 7 8 1 8 7 1 1 7 7 5 3 4 *